"In a world that complicates the most natural and pure things that we have like food and health care, this book delivers the straightforward, blockbuster formula that can cause the change that we each long for. Dr. Pfeiffer has proposed the immediate and profound actions that will deliver change as desired. To teachers like him we owe our freedom to live strong in an ailing world."

STUART WHITE
Director of Whole Health Associates Natural Healing Center, Houston, Texas

"Having worked with Dr. Pfeiffer professionally for over a decade, I can say, with no reservations, that he lives by the same principles he reveals in this book. His experience with thousands of patients, as well as his deep concern for their welfare, qualifies him to present this vital material. This book can be the beginning of a journey to a healthy life that is so elusive today."

BENTON E. WIGTON
President, Standard Process of PA, Inc.

"Those who search the pages of this book will find nothing but treasures and wisdom that can and will change their life and health as they know it. Dr Pfeiffer has hit it out of the park! Dr. Pfeiffer is a mentor to me and our missions are completely aligned. This book has the answers to a long, healthy, happy life. Dr. Pfeiffer is a passionate genius when it comes to knowledge and understanding of the human body. This book is a tell all to finding health and happiness!"

DAN HIGGINSON
Founder, CEO Synergy Worldwide

DR. PFEIFFER'S GUIDE TO A

LONGER
HEALTHIER LIFE

DR. PFEIFFER'S GUIDE TO A

LONGER
HEALTHIER LIFE

SIMPLE LIFESTYLE CHANGES

TO SET YOUR LIFE ON THE PATH TO

HEALTH AND WELLNESS

DOUGLAS G. PFEIFFER, D.C.

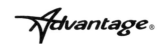

Published by Advantage, Charleston, South Carolina.
Member of Advantage Media Group.

ADVANTAGE is a registered trademark and the Advantage colophon is a trademark of Advantage Media Group, Inc.

Printed in the United States of America.

ISBN: 978-159932-271-1
LCCN: 2014954405

Book design by George Stevens.

This publication is designed to provide accurate and authoritative information in regard to the subject matter covered. It is sold with the understanding that the publisher is not engaged in rendering legal, accounting, or other professional services. If legal advice or other expert assistance is required, the services of a competent professional person should be sought.

Although the author and publisher have made every effort to ensure that the information in this book was correct at press time, the author and publisher do not assume and hereby disclaim any liability to any party for any loss, damage, or disruption caused by errors or omissions, whether such errors or omissions result from negligence, accident, or any other cause.

This book is not intended as a substitute for, and nothing contained in this book shall be construed or interpreted as, the medical advice of a licensed, practicing physician. The reader should regularly consult a physician in matters relating to his/her health and particularly with respect to any symptoms that may require diagnosis or medical attention.

Advantage Media Group is proud to be a part of the Tree Neutral® program. Tree Neutral offsets the number of trees consumed in the production and printing of this book by taking proactive steps such as planting trees in direct proportion to the number of trees used to print books. To learn more about Tree Neutral, please visit **www.treeneutral.com**. To learn more about Advantage's commitment to being a responsible steward of the environment, please visit **www.advantagefamily.com/green**

Advantage Media Group is a publisher of business, self-improvement, and professional development books and online learning. We help entrepreneurs, business leaders, and professionals share their Stories, Passion, and Knowledge to help others Learn & Grow. Do you have a manuscript or book idea that you would like us to consider for publishing? Please visit **advantagefamily.com** or call **1.866.775.1696.**

DEDICATION

When you stop to think about it, it's amazing how many people influence who you become and what you do in life. With that in mind, I must really go back to give credit where credit is due for this book and everything that lead up to its creation.

I would first like to thank God for the blessings and opportunities that have been placed before me. I truly appreciate the guidance and strength that my faith has given to me over the years.

It's taken five years, but I could not have completed this book or all of the other wonderful accomplishments of my life without the love, confidence, and support of my "Partner in Life", Liane. My wife has stood by me and kept the ship afloat through weekends and nights alone while I was hard at work at the office or writing this book. She has ensured that our two sons have all of the support they need to grow up well, despite their Dad's many long nights away. She is my toughest critic and my biggest supporter. Without Liane, none of this would have been possible.

To my Dad, I would like to posthumously thank you for the will of steel that you gave me to plow through any impediment that I encounter. Without that will, I would have given up on a lot of tasks, duties, and responsibilities that have shaped my life.

To my Mom, thank you for teaching me compassion. You showed me that success in life means a lot more than just a big bank account. You demonstrated to me that touching and improving people's lives is really what this journey is all about.

To everyone else who contributed to this work—from my mentors over the years to my family—thank you for everything that you have done to make this journey truly enjoyable. To my daughter-in-law, Suzanne, I appreciate your contributions, support, and assistance with editing. And Sabrina, thank you for enduring my deadlines and helping to research for this book. If we had been blessed with daughters, we would have prayed for them to be both of you.

TABLE OF CONTENTS

INTRODUCTION

"The doctor of the future will use no medicine but will interest his patients in the care of the human frame in diet and the cause and prevention of disease."

—THOMAS EDISON

hiropractic medicine has been around since 1895, but to many people it's still a new idea. I've been in practice for nearly 30 years, and I'm still asked what it was that originally drew me to chiropractic medicine. The fact that it was a drug-less healing profession was intriguing, and the philosophy of it made sense to me with my biology background, as did the physiology on which chiropractic is based.

Over the last 120 years, there has been a lot of economic, political, and medical animosity between the different schools of thought prevalent in the healing professions. To give you some perspective on our profession and how the medical establishment has tried and failed to shut it down: In the 1970s, a group of five chiropractors initiated a class-action suit against the American Medical Association (AMA). The AMA had formed the Anti-Quackery Commission, ostensibly to protect consumers from fraudulent medical practitioners, but its own internal memorandum revealed that the actual intention was to contain or eliminate the profession of chiropractic. Over the 11 years that followed, these five chiropractors won every case at every level up to the federal court. Ultimately, the AMA caved at the federal court level because it didn't want this case to go to the Supreme Court and, as a result, had to print retractions and pay restitution.

Historically, virtually every alternative health care profession has suffered similar attacks from the medical establishment. For example, homeopathy, which has recently seen resurgence both in the United States and abroad, was essentially eliminated in this country. At its inception in 1848, what would later come to be known as the Hahnemann Medical College in Philadelphia—now part of Drexel University—was intended to be a homeopathic hospital. Its founders, three homeopathic physicians who were influenced by Dr. Samuel Hahnemann (1755–1843), the German founder of homeopathy, used only homeopathic remedies[1]. Naturopathy was also effectively marginalized and eliminated. Osteopathy was originally an alternative form of medical treatment, first proposed in the 1850s by Andrew Taylor Still (1828–1917), a medical doctor who was disillusioned with the profession when he lost three of his children to spinal meningitis. He created the system of osteopathy, which was very similar to chiropractic, although they based their philosophy on the circulatory system

---

1   "History of the Institution: Untried and Alternative Paths in Medical Education," http:// archives.drexelmed.edu/history.php.

as opposed to the chiropractic profession's concentration on the nervous system. Ultimately, the medical establishment effectively absorbed the profession of osteopathy, so if you go to an osteopath today, you are essentially seeing a medical doctor.

Pretty much everybody else was pushed out of the path of economic competition with the medical establishment, except for chiropractic. They just could not get rid of us chiropractors, but that hasn't stopped them from trying. A lot of the things that you have probably heard over the years about chiropractors killing people or having poor education are just not factual. In fact, during *Wilk et al. v. the American Medical Association* (1990), researchers compared the cadaver dissection classes and course work at the University of Chicago Medical School with that at the National College of Chiropractic, which is located in Lombard, Illinois, right outside of Chicago. The studies indicated that the chiropractic classes on those subjects were equal, or superior in some respects, to the medical education in these classes that was received at the University of Chicago Medical School.

In the quote at the beginning of this chapter, Thomas Edison is saying that the future of medicine will rely on natural methods of health care, and that's an accurate summation of what we do. The education that we receive in nutrition is thorough and in many respects superior to what's offered in medical schools, especially considering the fact that most medical schools offer little or no training in nutrition or other natural health care methods.

I see many other physical and physiological changes in patients who come into my office for a condition that chiropractors commonly treat, like back pain, neck pain, or headaches. We see so many other functions in patients' body systems improving as a result of being adjusted. This is without even adding in nutritional counseling, supplementation, or the other components that I feel strongly must be incorporated into a holistic health care paradigm.

Why have I taken time from my already busy schedule to write this book? I've given a lot of thought to the question of why I ended up where I am, doing what I'm doing. When I think back on it, I was always interested in biology. I used to like to study animals. When I was a kid, I would bring home dead animals that I had found to study (much to my mother's chagrin) because I wanted to know how their bodies functioned. I learned compassion through living with a mother who suffered from depression, although her condition probably wasn't completely diagnosed back then. It gave me an innate understanding of people's emotions and feelings, which allowed me to build the practice that I have today. In supporting her emotionally, I felt responsible for helping her to have a better day, so to speak.

As I grew up, I developed the understanding that the body needs to be nurtured and taken care of, and that it should be maintained in as pure an environment as possible. My mom was a smoker, and one of the things that I nagged her about incessantly was quitting. Even though I was just an eight-year-old kid, I came up with all kinds of ploys and tricks to get her to stop, including taking her cigarettes and hiding them. I remember one birthday gift I got for her was a cigarette dispenser in the form of a miniature coffin. You put the cigarettes in it, then when you pressed a button, a skeletal hand would come out and hand you one. Not exactly subtle, but it got my message across. The impetus to relentlessly nurturing healthful lifestyle changes in others was sparked by childhood experiences such as these.

More than ever, I feel the need to educate people as well as heal them. Education has always been a critical component of my mantra and my practice. There are things that people don't understand, and if you can clarify these health-related concepts and assist them in making concurrent lifestyle changes, it really turns the light on for them. I want to help others grasp this revolutionary philosophy and how it applies to health and health care. I want you to know how simple it is to make small changes that can have an enormous positive effect in your life, not only on your health, but also in your interaction with others.

CHAPTER 1

THE PROBLEM OF CONVENTIONAL THINKING

"Conventional wisdom says such discoveries should not be happening now."

—ANONYMOUS

Our notions about health, and by extension the design of our health care delivery system, are largely based on the idea that illness is something that simply happens to us, or something that we're predisposed to because of our genetic makeup; in short, something over which we have no real control. Thus, our health care system is largely dedicated to putting out fires, rather than preventing them. But your own good sense and observation should tell you that, in this case, conventional wisdom has it wrong. We aren't helpless, and our bodies aren't our enemies. On the contrary, what we do and how we think about working with, rather than against, our bodies, must be part of the paradigmatic shift we need to make if we're to move toward wellness and away from disease.

Our health care costs are going up exponentially and, in my opinion, unnecessarily, because of what we do to ourselves and thereby to our health as a result. We will see that our disease and sickness costs will continue to spiral out of control in the future if we don't make some changes in our individual and collective lifestyles. These changes are not difficult to make, but they are essential to our survival as individuals, as a society, and as a world. Unfortunately, our world is going down the wrong path. The disease and sickness paradigm is not where true health is to be found. We must shift paths to the health and wellness paradigm or we will continue down the same path of preventable, chronic, debilitating diseases and disorders.

I'm a strong advocate of understanding degenerative conditions like Alzheimer's. Both my grandfather and my father had Alzheimer's, so that doesn't bode well for me. But if we could just get beyond the limitations of our cultural thinking medically and societally about Alzheimer's and move forward with some common-sense alternative approaches to this devastating disorder, we would make dramatic change in its progression.

In much of what I'm going to discuss with you, you'll notice that I don't refer to a lot of conditions of modern society as diseases, including cancer, because I don't believe that they are specific disease entities in and of themselves. I feel that they are disorders, not diseases.

Take Alzheimer's, for instance. In the brain, individuals affected with Alzheimer's develop amyloid plaques. For years, the belief has been that the amyloid plaques were actually the cause of the problem. For lack of a better description, they're like congealed gunk in your brain composed of a number of proteins and minerals that we thought were blockades to nerve impulses in the brain.

A pharmaceutical company recently developed a drug that would actually dissolve or break down amyloid plaques, and those researchers were thinking: "Great. We'll get rid of the plaques, and then there will be normal synapses." (Synapses are areas between nerves in the brain across which nerve impulses must travel.) In other words, there would be normal nerve transmission in the brain and everything would be good. The company was on the third, or tertiary, phase of testing, which was where they used the drug on the public in a controlled setting. They found that the subjects who were taking the drug that dissolved these plaques actually got worse. Their Alzheimer's progressed at a more rapid rate than those individuals who were taking a placebo. Subsequently, they stopped the study, scrapping this multimillion-dollar product they had been developing and said, "We've got to start over. We have to rethink this whole amyloid plaque thing; maybe these plaques are not the cause of the problem. Maybe they are actually protecting the brain in some way."

That discovery brings us full circle to why I got into chiropractic. Rather than trying to outthink the body and assuming we know better, we need to recognize that the body is amazing in its capabilities, in what it can do, and how it can do it. If the body is creating amyloid plaques, it's got to be doing it for a reason. *There is nothing the body does that's wrong.* Everything it does is right. Circumstances and the situation that cause it to do something or react in a certain way may be wrong, but what it's doing is right in response to the circumstances. If the body's creating amyloid plaques in the brain, we shouldn't be looking at getting rid of those amyloid plaques without first ascertaining their function. Maybe we should stop doing what has created the necessity for the body to develop these plaques to protect us. Perhaps we've created these circumstances through our lifestyle, through our choices, and through our decisions about what we do with and to ourselves on a daily basis.

In medicine, we try to label something as a disease, and typically, we do that because we either have already developed or are in the process of developing a drug for it. I raise a lot of eyebrows when I make that comment above about cancer. But how much progress have we actually made in dealing with this condition? In the 1700s, the treatment for breast cancer was to remove the breast. Fast-forward 250 years; one of our treatments is often to still remove the breast. We've added a number of other things like radiation and chemo, but ultimately, we're often just going to excise the damaged tissue.

I do not believe that cancer is a disease. I believe that cancer is a symptom of something that's gone wrong or is out of balance in the body, and it's the body's way of dealing with it. What changes those specific cells and triggers them to mutate and begin to multiply in an unnatural and unhealthy way? If we have a condition that we've been affected by for hundreds of years, and its ultimate treatment, at least in the last 200 years, is largely the same, and the incidence of this condition or disorder is climbing, then something must be wrong with the way in which we are approaching the condition. We need to consider changing the way we are thinking about and dealing with this devastating condition.

The medical pharmaceutical world is based on selling drugs. The pharmaceutical industry is marketing its product, drugs, in ways it couldn't have done 20 years ago. Today, the US Food and Drug Administration (FDA) allows the marketing of drugs on television and radio; people will now go to a doctor's office and suggest that they be prescribed a particular drug. Drugs are necessary and helpful for many people, but the more people on the drugs, the more money pharmaceutical companies make. My goal with the services and educational programs I provide is to assist my patients and the public in using safer alternatives when possible.

Life expectancy over the last 100 years has increased significantly.

Today, our average life span is 78 years. If we look at statistics, the number of individuals living to age 90 and beyond has tripled in the last three decades to 2 million people. The number of individuals surviving to age 90 and above by 2050 will quadruple, but the questions remain: Are we living better? Are we living healthier? The answer is that we're absolutely not. All we need to observe is the quality of life, particularly in the second half of our lives.

Nearly all of those living in nursing homes have one or more disabilities, and 80 percent of those who are not in a nursing facility have a disability. Five million Americans today suffer from Alzheimer's disease, according to the National Institutes of Health. By 2050, even if we have major treatment breakthroughs, 16 million people will develop Alzheimer's. Look at what that's going to do to our society relative to medical costs: $1 trillion dollars a year to treat those people. We've created a society in which medical expenses for drugs, surgery, and medical care go up exponentially as we age to the point where, statistically, in the last six months of an individual's life, they will incur as much or more in medical expenses than they have their entire life to that point.

I had a patient in my office who couldn't stand up straight and who was hospitalized twice because of this. She had no insurance, and I hate to think what her bill for those hospitalizations must have been. I treated her *once*, and she was able to walk out of my office erect and under her own power. There's something wrong with this picture. This is an indication of a system that is broken, and we, the health care consuming community, must take the responsibility to fix it. It is possible to change this system. Our health care system is consumer driven. As a patient can dictate to the doctor which drug to prescribe, you too have a great deal of power over the medical system. The system is changing, but the changes are dangerously slow. It's kind of like turning an oil tanker around. Those goliaths don't turn on a dime, and neither will the health care delivery system. It will take time, energy, and a concerted effort.

That's really the reason I'm so passionate about this subject and have been my entire life. I always felt that the body had the ability to heal itself given the proper circumstances. We can assist the body in making the shift toward health and wellness at any point, but the earlier you start, the easier it is. We have to look at not just adding years to our lives, but also at the flip side, what I describe as adding life to those years. People need to know that there are things that can be done to deter, eliminate, or at least significantly slow the progress or onset of some of these debilitating diseases and disorders. As I often say in my seminars and to my patients, diabetes is the most easily preventable disorder that we have, yet it leads to virtually every other disease or disorder that people die from. These diabetes-related conditions take the form of cancer and kidney failure, as well as heart attacks and strokes.

Another problem that's looming on the public health horizon is the rising incidence of metabolic syndrome. What is metabolic syndrome? For starters, you need to know that a syndrome is just a group of signs and symptoms that, taken together, appear in a segment of the population. Health care researchers and providers look at that and say, "Okay. This is a group of things that a lot of people have, so we're going to label it and call it a syndrome." That applies not only to metabolic syndrome but also to fibromyalgia syndrome, chronic fatigue syndrome, and many other syndromes. These are conditions that no one can necessarily label with any clarity and say, "This is what causes it." It's not like there's a particular bacteria that brings it on. But there are a lot of people who share these signs and symptoms, so it is labeled as a syndrome.

What is metabolic syndrome? I'll go into a discussion at length about it later, but briefly, it boils down to the body's inability to use food and food products (I'll define that one later, too) that are consumed. From a medical standpoint, the components of metabolic syndrome are obesity (significantly overweight, which applies to most Americans), insulin resistance (prediabetes), dyslipidemia (generally elevated cholesterol levels), and hypertension (high blood pressure). What does that mean? Metabolic syndrome causes you to get fat, particularly around the waist; you develop high cholesterol, high blood sugar, and high blood pressure.

We have drugs that will treat high blood pressure. We have drugs that will treat high blood sugar. We have drugs that will treat high cholesterol. We haven't quite perfected the class of drugs to successfully treat obesity yet, but it is being worked on. The problem is that you can take all of those drugs and you'll still have metabolic syndrome; ultimately, metabolic syndrome develops from poor lifestyle choices that lead to what's called insulin resistance and a plethora of other conditions that are secondary to metabolic syndrome. One of the causes of this is that you have shoved so much sugar into your body and bloodstream that your natural supply of insulin, which is produced by your pancreas and allows sugar to go into the cells, isn't sufficient to handle the job.

For the Paleolithic man, that was very important because he only ate once every two or three days, so the paleo man needed to be able to store some of that food. It was necessary to physically store it to eat later or burn later when it was needed. Your liver will convert unused sugar to fat, store it, and then, when it's time, create a hormone that will break it down into sugar again. That way you can use it when you need it.

Why doesn't it work that way for us today? Because we keep putting more sugar into our systems; excessive fat is created as a result, and because there's no place else to put it, the body stockpiles it around our belly, hips, thighs, legs, and arms. Sadder still is the part of this we can't see: excess fat is being stored inside of your body as well—gobbets of fat are being piled on and in your organs.

When I was in my human dissection lab at Palmer College of Chiropractic in Davenport, Iowa, I was amazed when we dissected the abdomen and chest of an obese female cadaver that we were working on. It was an eye opener for me to see the fatty masses encapsulating this poor women's heart, kidneys, and virtually all of her internal organs. Imagine how hard it was for those organs to perform their duties every day with the extra coating of fat on them. It would be like trying to run a marathon with three sweaters, two overcoats, ski pants over your jeans, and heavy winter snow boots on. The liver will store the fat inside itself, too, so you end up with the latest disease in the medical world, fatty liver disease, which is the leading cause of cirrhosis of the liver.

All of this is preventable. Drugs are not the answer. The answer is to change what caused the problem: what goes into our mouths; our lack of physical activity; our hyperactive, stressed-out lives; and our lack of quality sleep. These lifestyle abnormalities create the environment for insulin resistance and all of the other components of metabolic syndrome. The way you are going to change what caused the problem is to get rid of the high sugar levels, start moving your body more, learn how to modify your stress levels, and get quality healthful sleep. If you do that, you will rid yourself of the components of metabolic syndrome.

As you can see, we need to reboot our thinking about health and wellness. Diabetes is the most preventable disorder in our culture, yet there are millions of people who are taking diabetic drugs and doing nothing to change what's causing that diabetes.

It's not their fault. It is really a lack of knowledge and ignorance about this subject. They don't understand what they need to do, and they're so hooked on the wrong things that it's difficult to make the change.

At the Center for Nutrition and Wellness, our philosophy is that there are four pillars to health: eat right, sleep right, think right, and move right. One of the biggest things that we do in our practice is change people's lifestyle, yet it is one of the most difficult things to accomplish. Mass marketing has made it too easy to get kids hooked on soda, on Twinkies, on you-name-it. That's causing the problem, not that we don't have enough glipizide or metformin in our bloodstream.

We don't eat right, and we certainly don't think right, sleep right, or move right. We must think about stress in a new light and how it physiologically changes our bodies later in life. We all know that we don't move around enough. We're sedentary when we should be moving throughout the day. We don't sleep right. We live in the most sleep-deprived society, and we pay for that with the physiological changes that occur as a result of our fatigue and sleep deprivation. Your likelihood of developing diabetes increases when you're sleep deprived, as does the incidence of Alzheimer's disease.

The question becomes, not "Is there a problem?" but "What can we do about it?" In the next chapter, we'll address this question.

CHAPTER 2

THE HEALTH AND WELLNESS PARADIGM

"The greatest wealth is health."

—VIRGIL

I n my experience, I find that individuals react very enthusiastically to the idea of being healthy and well. Unfortunately, because of how our culture and our socioeconomic medical system work, we live in a crisis care system. We are used to waiting for things to erupt, and then dealing with them. The other unfortunate truth is that our current crisis care system is not the true health and wellness paradigm that I am referring to.

An example I often use with patients to make this point about true prevention and health and wellness is a colonoscopy. We currently look at a colonoscopy as a preventative procedure. We also look at a mammogram as a preventative procedure. But if we truly use the word as it is defined and as it's intended to be used, they're not preventative. To prevent something means to keep it from occurring. The two procedures that I am using as examples here are really early detection procedures to find a problem that's already there. If you have a colonoscopy and your colon is perfectly clean and everything is good, then the doctor may say: "Great, we'll do another one in five years." What have you actually prevented?

So we wait. Every day you continue to do the same things, which are often the wrong things relative to your overall health and wellness. You don't change anything in your lifestyle as a result of the findings of your colonoscopy. In five years, you get checked again to see if you've developed a polyp or colon cancer. Now, don't get me wrong; if they discover and remove a polyp that is pre-cancerous, it's a good thing, but you are doing nothing to correct what caused that polyp or cancer to develop in the intervening five years.

It's the same thing with a mammogram. Mammograms are routinely recommended as a preventive procedure. However, if your mammogram is clear, you're still going to have another mammogram in a year, two years, or even five years later. If you have a mammogram that detects something, you may have a biopsy or a needle biopsy to see if that lump or calcification detected on the mammogram is actually cancer. Again, it may be an effective early detection procedure, but it's certainly not preventing anything. True prevention is taking corrective action by altering the things you do day in and day out in your lifestyle. It's through those changes that you can positively affect your duration of life, your quality of life, and your ability to avoid the things that we look at today as almost inevitable disorders.

As the costs of our current health care delivery system spiral out of control, we are looking for techniques and procedures to be the most cost effective as well as the most beneficial for patients. If we were to look at true preventative techniques as an alternative to our current crisis management mentality, it would create significant reductions in health care costs.

We talked a little bit about Alzheimer's disease. If we were to proactively look at the things that can be done today to retard the progression or avoid the onset of Alzheimer's disease, we would save trillions of dollars in health care costs in the coming decades. And they're very simple things; for example, increasing vitamin D intake, taking omega-3 fish oil, and eating vegetables and fruits. By taking actions as easy as these, you can prevent or retard the onset of a condition that's as devastating as Alzheimer's disease.

The best way to prevent colon cancer is to change what is going into the pipes, so to speak. If you put in the food that you are genetically designed to eat, rather than the things we have created (what I always call "product" as opposed to "food"), you will significantly reduce your potential of getting colon cancer. Imagine that, reducing the incidence of the second-leading cause of cancer deaths in the United States today.

What are the current treatment techniques that our disease and sickness care system uses to deal with something like colon cancer? Basically, it boils down to three approaches. One is surgery; we cut it out. Two is radiation; we burn it out. Three is chemotherapy; we alter the chemistry of the cells. It's unfortunate because both radiation and chemotherapy actually can cause cancer.

We'll talk more extensively about genetic predisposition to disorders and diseases like cancer or Alzheimer's. There are, however, some revealing research studies that have been performed with identical twins who both have the BRCA2 gene, which predisposes them to breast cancer. One twin gets breast cancer and one does not. If the genetic theory holds true, they both should have breast cancer. Clearly, there are things above and beyond genetics that affect these disorders. Most of these variables relate to whether or not we are creating an environment that allows the cells and tissues in this ecosystem we call our bodies to proliferate, grow, and survive for an extended period of time. Bodies are designed to last much longer than they do.

SUFFICIENCY AND PURITY

If we want to live not only longer but also better, we must create an environment for this ecosystem that creates both *sufficiency* and *purity*. A mentor of mine, Dr. James Chestnut, introduced these terms to me. A pioneer in the health and wellness field, Dr. Chestnut changed my views about health and health care and sent me down a path of study that has allowed me to create a holistic health and wellness center, The Center for Nutrition and Wellness, based not only on his teachings but also on those of other great practitioners in the field like Jeffery Bland, PhD; Andrew Weil, MD; Robert Atkins, MD; and many others.

So what do these two words mean in the practical sense? Sufficiency is, obviously, giving the body what it needs in sufficient quantity and quality to proliferate and grow and to maintain and sustain. We want good, quality food going into our body, as one example. But we want good, quality information going into our body, too.

We want good, quality thoughts because when we look at the concept of sufficiency, it goes across the spectrum of our health paradigm from eating right to thinking right. It's about much more than food; we are looking at the four pillars of health as those things that we want in sufficiency and purity. We want not only our food, but also our thoughts to be sufficient and of good quality. We are discovering the relationship between the mind and the body in so many more ways. We want to nurture that aspect of our health and wellness paradigm as well.

The definition of *sufficiency* is *enough*. We want enough of the things that are necessary to be healthy and well. We want enough vitamin D, omega-3 fatty acids, and enough B vitamins going into our system. Unfortunately, the diets that we have today are significantly deficient in most, if not all, of those necessary requirements for health and wellness.

Purity, however, looks to the quality of those things. If we examine the purity of our foodstuffs, we will recognize the potential effect that things such as genetically modified foods have on our overall health and wellness. We then begin to recognize that the purity of the substances we are taking in is critical. There are studies that have been done on fetal umbilical blood samples that show that the fetuses already have levels of pesticides and other environmental chemicals in their bloodstreams. The environmental aspects of our food sources, our air, and our water are critical.

When I look at this paradigm of health and wellness and sufficiency and purity, I feel that we are not only polluting our environment and ecosystem externally, but we are also polluting our environment and ecosystem internally. Our bodies are becoming more and more toxic. We need to consider that aspect of health and wellness when we look at what changes we may need to make, not only as individuals but also as a society, to clean our bodies and our environment.

What is genetically modified food? Let's take corn for an example, because it's a dietary staple in our society (although it shouldn't be, but we will discuss that a little later). Most of the corn we produce in the United States is genetically modified; we implant a gene into corn that is resistant to herbicides. That means the farmer can use all of the herbicide he wants around that plant and the corn will be resistant to it, but all of the weeds around it will be killed off. The fact is that we don't understand how ingesting that modified genetic material may affect us, which is why many European countries have banned genetically modified foods. That certainly is not the way that food was designed to be, and we're creating something new without knowing what harm it may cause us.

Another thing to consider when assessing the purity of our foods is our soil quality. Because our soil is nutrient-deficient, when we grow vegetables, the nutrients they get are coming primarily from the fertilizer that is used, which is nitrogen-based. We have depleted our soil of minerals and other valuable nutrients that would have been taken up by those plants and passed along to us when we consumed those crops. Instead, we have supplanted those nutrients with nitrogen, which allows the plant to grow, but it doesn't give it any significant nutritional value above and beyond what it can scrape from the soil itself. To make things worse, the runoff from that nitrogen-based fertilizer goes into our oceans and is now creating dead zones in the oceans where nothing can survive. We've created an industrial farming base in the United States that is only interested in the quantity of food that can be produced to obtain the biggest amount of money in return.

Compare that to where we were 150 years ago when we lived in a small farm-based country, in communities where people were growing food in nutrient-rich soil. Let's correlate that with the duration and quality of life that those individuals experienced, taking into consideration that there were other hardships that they experienced that we don't necessarily contend with today. If we restrict our conversation to just the foods that they took in and the nutrients that they received from them, those folks lived a lot healthier lifestyles and their lives ended the way they were designed to. They did not deteriorate over a 20-year period; they lived productively right up until their last days, then they died in their sleep. They didn't waste away and gradually decline mentally and physically over a 10-, 15-, or 20-year period. What we must strive for is the paradigm of our ancestors who ate wholesome, real foods that they raised themselves. Those ancestors also received sound, sufficient sleep and moved throughout their day. They had the normal worries of life, but didn't have the stress-filled lives that many of us lead today. In other words, they lived lives that were more genetically congruent.

TOXICITY AND DEFICIENCY

Now, let's look at toxicity and deficiency (also terms first coined in this context by my mentor Dr. James Chestnut). We live in an extremely toxic environment. Part of that is caused by industrial pollution, but it also involves the things that we do ourselves every day. We drink chlorinated water, for example. We chlorinate water on a large-scale basis in communities to create drinking water that is potable and will not cause disease. However, when we put this quantity of chlorine in the water that we drink, that amount of chlorine can create other health problems. For example, we have a significant iodine deficiency in our society.

In the 1920s and 1930s, the federal government began to require iodizing of salt because large numbers of people, particularly in the Midwest (the bread basket), were developing goiters, which is an enlargement of the thyroid gland due to insufficient iodine in the soil to support the thyroid glands in the general population. Because the soils were iodine deficient and the plants couldn't get iodine from these depleted soils, we didn't get it in our food sources. The US government deemed it necessary to iodize something that everyone consumed, and so salt was chosen. Understand, though, that the quantity of iodine mandated to be used in iodized salt was just enough to keep the population from developing a goiter, not necessarily enough to create sufficiency of iodine in the human body.

With the chlorination of water, the problem is that chlorine, along with bromine and fluorine, are competitive binders for iodine. In other words, if you don't have sufficient iodine in your system, chlorine, fluorine, and bromine will bind to sites on the thyroid and other glands in the body. Unfortunately, chlorine can't perform the same duties that the iodine would, so we start having other problems due to this deficiency, which will later be diagnosed as disease. This is one reason why we have such significantly high incidences of thyroid problems in our culture; many people are significantly iodine deficient because we are supplanting our iodine with chlorine, bromine, and fluorine.

The problems arising from the widespread fluoridation of our public water supplies are another example of a toxicity syndrome. Fluorine and fluoride were industrial byproducts from the aluminum manufacturing industry. In the 1940s and 1950s, it was decided that this industrial byproduct should be used as an additive in our drinking water because it was purported to be beneficial for the general population's teeth. Today, the quantity of fluoride that we are using in our public water supply is being revaluated. The US Food and Drug Administration is making alterations to the recommended amounts of fluoride being added to drinking water because it is seeing the detrimental effects on dental enamel resulting from the high quantity of added fluoride in drinking water. These examples are typical of the unintended consequences that can occur when we try to solve one problem and inadvertently create another.

Deficiency is obvious and attributable to the degree that we're eating product rather than food. By *product*, I mean man-made things. I say to my patients, "Anything that you find in the center of a supermarket is going to be product." Anything you find around the periphery, in most cases, is going to be food, because that's where they keep the vegetables, the fruits, the meats, and the dairy. If you eat from the center of the supermarket—if you eat processed food, if you eat fast food, as some people do as a routine diet—you're getting little to no nutrition, other than salt, fat, and simple carbohydrates that are converted to sugar very rapidly. This plays into why and how we create some diseases and disorders that we again consider just routine things that "we are all going to end up with."

Diabetes is an example. We load our systems with sugar and then wonder why we end up with diabetes. The deficit of good, quality nutritious food and nutrients going into our ecosystem, which we call our body, creates that deficiency. Sure, we have plenty of product, but we don't have a lot of food going into our bodies, so we create a scenario where those products create nutritional deficiencies.

Certainly there are choices that we all have to make. One of my frustrations in my practices is compliance. That's a frustration with any physician today, because patients' compliance is out of the doctor's control. Insurance companies are all over that too. If a patient is not compliant, they need to be discharged according to insurance company guidelines. For a patient to be compliant with the paradigm that I live and profess to them, they have to change their belief system. They have to live outside of the conventional world.

My family and I have been doing this for 30 years. It's not an easy thing to do sometimes because you are looked at as being different. On many occasions, I've been accused by my sons of being a buzz kill, because I don't eat the pizza at a ball game or the snacks at a Super Bowl party. Admittedly, it's tough for folks to make that jump. If they do, even temporarily, it's difficult for them to stay there. The pace of life we have sometimes necessitates or at least creates the illusion that it's necessary that we do these things. It certainly isn't, but we believe the fallacy that it is.

One of my goals with my patients is to help them understand that that's not necessary. I feel strongly that you can't force a patient or an individual to make that transition. They have to be ready, willing, and able to make it. The lifestyle changes that we incorporate into people's lives unquestionably can and do make a huge difference in their overall health and wellness as well as their overall longevity. It's a no-brainer; a lot of what I'm going to discuss in this book sounds simple, because it *is* simple, but it's not easy to do. If you can make those changes, you can create an environment in which your life, health, and body will change.

I tell folks when they go through our Full System Detox Cleanse Program that our intention is to change their lives when they exit this program. Once your brain is expanded to a different size and dimension, it will never return to where it was. If together we can make those belief system changes in a three-week period, you will not go back to where you were. That is my ultimate goal.

I always say I wear three hats in my practice. I'm certainly a doctor first, but I am also a coach as well as a teacher. The word doctor came from the Latin word meaning *to teach*. Part of my job as a healer is to teach my patients, and I strive to do that with each and every one of them. While there is a great deal of personal responsibility required on their part, in the initial phases some of it is a shared responsibility, because you do need a teacher to guide you along this difficult and challenging path.

CHAPTER 3

EAT RIGHT

"Life is not merely being alive, but being well."

~MARCUS VALERIUS MARTIALIS

I n the last chapter, we introduced the idea of toxicity and deficiency. I spoke about the toxins, but I did not speak about toxicity of quantity. If we look at what I am referring to as toxicity, you will see that you can have a toxicity of virtually anything; even a toxicity of water going into your system. You can certainly have a toxicity of food, which most people in this country do. To put it plainly, we eat too much.

There are numerous studies that show that by restricting our caloric intake we can extend our lives significantly. One study showed that by reducing our caloric intake by one-third we could extend our lifespan by 20 percent. If your current habits mean that you'll live to age 70, you would live to 84 if you just ate less food.

Now, that is an amazing finding. It sets a clear goal that should be easily attainable. If people simply looked ahead, they would see that following this advice could allow them to enjoy 14 more years of quality life. Imagine 14 more years of time to spend with your children and grandchildren, or to enjoy golf, or to pass along more family stories and history to the next two generations. You would also be able to be productive and contribute to society, rather than being a drain on your family and society. Again, the choice requires taking personal responsibility, not just with you in mind but for the good of others, too. Unfortunately, for most of us, it isn't quite as easy as it sounds.

The toxicity in our diets that we're talking about has been created by numerous factors. Some of those factors are very difficult to correct because of some of the things our society does, like fluoridating water. I realize that for many individuals reading this book, the concept of not having fluoride treatments on their teeth or fluoridation of their water may sound absurd. But the fact is that by attempting to engineer our health with the use of food additives, we're creating diets that are genetically incongruent with the way we were designed to live.

We do not require fluoride to be added to our diets for us to be healthy. When we begin eating right, we have sufficient calcium and other minerals going into our system to have strong, healthy teeth. When our diet is genetically incongruent, our way of thinking dictates that we make up the deficiencies with additives in an attempt to fix what wasn't broken. The issue is that this kind of tinkering doesn't work, and it ultimately creates more problems than it solves.

A generational study was done in the 1930s by Dr. Francis M. Pottinger Jr. Dr. Pottinger's study was performed on cats. In this study, he fed the cats one of three diets. The first group was fed what was genetically congruent for a cat to eat: raw meat and raw milk. The second group got a diet of cooked meat and condensed milk, and the third group was fed cooked meat and evaporated milk. While the first group developed normally, the latter two groups in this study ended up developing all sorts of changes and mutations in their systems as a result of what they were eating.

Those conditions that Dr. Pottinger's cats developed were the same diseases of our modern society. Their offspring started to get sicker and sicker. Their lifespans shortened, and ultimately, they got to the point where they were infertile. They had hair loss, they lost their teeth, and the structure of their skeletons changed, all within seven generations. We have been doing what we are doing now in our food supply for close to that long generationally as humans. By the seventh generation, those cats could not come back. In other words, even if that seventh generation of sick, infertile, disease-ridden cats had begun to eat the way they were genetically designed to eat, they could not have become healthy. They were societal wreckage, born without a chance at health.

I don't drink coffee, but we need to wake up and smell the coffee because we're getting to the point of no return. What sort of conditions do we have now that we didn't have years ago? Obviously, socially there were a lot of things we didn't discuss years ago, but I know many of these conditions did not occur years ago as they do today, like the infertility rates that we have today or erectile dysfunction, and Asperger syndrome (and is this truly a disease or a condition of our lifestyles?). When we think about the whole toxicity issue, we need to look at it generationally, because there is definitely a carryover from generation to generation.

We need to look at what is genetically congruent with our bodies and our genetic code, and the way we were designed to live our lives. Different animals are designed to eat and do different things. Look at our domestic animals; what does their food contain? Dog food typically contains corn, rice, and other grains. Dogs don't eat corn and rice in their natural environment; they eat meat. They have canine teeth to rip it apart. Now, look at what's happening to our pet cats and dogs. They are developing the same conditions, diseases, and disorders that we have: diabetes, heart disease, strokes, obesity, and epilepsy. I have patients who come into my office and tell me, "My cat has diabetes." or "My cat has epilepsy." It's just crazy, and here is the real clincher: They are put on the same drugs for those conditions that our current medical system provides in larger doses to us every year.

The food chain has essentially broken down. We are consuming both plant and animal products that, 150 years ago, were raised in a different way than they are today. As a result, we're changing. Today we see young girls reaching puberty at a much earlier age than they did 30 or 40 years ago. One significant cause for this is the bovine growth hormones that these girls inadvertently consume in meat and milk as they are growing up. These hormonal additives are being fed to cattle and dairy herds to spur their growth and production so that the producers can get their hormone- and antibiotic-laden meat product to market faster and make more money.

Not only is the meat stuffed with things you don't want (toxicity), but it's also poor in the nutrients (deficiency) you do want, things like good, healthy omega-3 fatty acids. We used to get omega-3s from the meat we consumed because that meat animal consumed grass, and grass is where the omega-3s came from. Today, cattle are raised on grains in feedlots. Grains are high in omega-6 fatty acids. This creates another toxicity issue because, in general, we are toxic in omega-6 fatty acids and we are deficient in omega-3 fatty acids because of what we're eating. The effects of this toxicity and deficiency are rampant.

In addition to the decrease in the age at which both male and female children reach puberty, we see the effects of these hormone-laden foods in rising rates of breast cancer, heart disease, and diabetes. If we look at the hormones that are used to fatten up and mature cattle and pigs, the hormone types oftentimes are estrogenic in their effects. Estrogen in certain forms precipitates the onset of cancer. It also acts to magnify the adverse effect that cancer has on our bodies. In other words, it causes the process to occur at a greater and faster rate.

The way the food that we are growing and processing affects us and has affected us generationally is becoming a greater concern not only here at home, but globally as well. Another example of a food product that we should discuss is margarine. Margarine was invented during World War II because we needed something to replace butter. The food scientists started with vegetable oil. They determined that if hydrogen was bubbled through the liquid vegetable (usually corn oil at the time) they could create a new food product that had a consistency and flavor similar to butter. It lacked the buttery color, so the food scientists simply added a packet of yellow powder that the consumer could mix into the pasty product. But just what is margarine? Well, it's a trans fat or a hydrogenated vegetable oil. You may recall that these are the substances that were outlawed in New York City restaurants. And why were they outlawed? Because they create significant adverse health consequences.

Fats are used in our body for many things, including every single wrapper or membrane around the cells in our bodies. Every cell has a membrane that is made using fat. If we incorporate these trans fats into that membrane, they become less permeable. This means that they don't allow things to go in and out very readily. This is in sharp contrast to the way normal lipid or fat wrappers for your cells work. In effect, we've created a barrier for the cells and made it more difficult for them to do their normal jobs.

The effects of all of this are that we've once again created both toxicities and deficiencies in our bodies with significant negative effects. I see the evidence of these effects in my patients every day. To reverse them, what we do in my office and what you must do in your life is to take baby steps. In my office, I have our patients do one thing at a time, and as we incorporate one thing, they begin to see the positive changes. This motivates them, as it will you, to do more to change their health and lives for the better.

For example, I had a patient who had very dry, scaly skin, which is one of the telltale signs of a deficiency in omega-3 fatty acids. On my recommendation, she started using the omega-3s. When I saw her again, I noticed that her skin was very moist and supple and no longer flaking. That success motivated her to make the effort to make the next positive change. Results are how we build on this whole health and wellness paradigm for patients, one that makes them say, "Hey, this looks good. I can see the change. I am losing some pounds." or "I am feeling better, so this must work." They get it, and then we can move on to the next thing to be corrected.

IS CHOLESTEROL THE ENEMY?

> *"The longer I live the less confidence I have in drugs and the greater is my confidence in the regulation and administration of diet and regimen."*
>
> —JOHN REDMAN COXE, 1800

We have been educated to think that cholesterol is a bad thing, and we want to drive the levels down as low as we can. Previously, the idea had been to drive the total cholesterol levels down to 200 or below. Now the medical establishment is shooting even lower, with 100 in some instances being the goal. What is the deal with this whole cholesterol thing?

First of all, keep in mind the concept that the body doesn't do anything wrong. Everything the body does is right. It may be trying to correct for something in some way. It could be trying to correct for something we've done wrong. Perhaps it is trying to correct for something that we put into it or something environmental over which we have little control. If we look at why cholesterol is there and what it's used for, we come to realize that it is not the enemy, but is actually an essential hormone in our bodies.

It's a fundamental building block for multiple other substances; for example, the sex hormones: estrogen, testosterone, and progesterone. Cholesterol is used by the body to manufacture these, as well as many stress hormones. It's used in the healing process when we are injured. It oftentimes is used to compensate for inflammation in an area of the body that is irritated and swollen. We incorporate cholesterol to sooth or protect an area that's inflamed. Remember what our parents would suggest to us when we were kids and burned ourselves? Put butter on the burn. The idea is the same when we look at the healing properties of cholesterol.

Inflammation is a significant negative health factor in our bodies, and we frequently create that inflammation by what we do. For example, if we look at arteries that are injured or damaged, one of the early components of that injury is inflammation in the lining of the artery. What the body does to help protect or soothe that area is to lay down some cholesterol-laden fatty tissue to soothe the artery's lining. Over time, because we don't do anything to correct the cause of this problem (which continues to create more inflammation), the body continues to lay down this fatty cholesterol-laden material in an attempt to soothe the injured lining of the artery. This attempt to heal the injured and inflamed tissue lining the artery ultimately forms a plaque or a blockage.

It is critical to understand that the body's laying down this cholesterol patch is not the bad thing. The cholesterol is something your body is trying to use to heal the bad thing; for example, the inflammation and the irritation in the lining of that artery. This applies to other areas in the body as well. Your body uses cholesterol in a good and appropriate way to remedy something that's gone wrong in the body. So why is it that we look at cholesterol as a bad substance in our bodies?

If I wanted to be cynical about it, I could point out that we have drugs now that will drive our cholesterol levels down artificially and get it into a lower range. The more people we have using those drugs, the more money the drug companies make. The medical profession has classified cholesterol as either good or bad. HDL cholesterol is medically labeled as good cholesterol, and LDL cholesterol is medically labeled as bad cholesterol, but these distinctions are neither accurate nor fair. Cholesterol is not good or bad; it's just appropriate to our body's needs.

One of the things that we don't even look at, which drives our cholesterol up, is stress in our lives. We'll talk about this in more detail later, but it's worth noting that our bodies are designed to sustain stress on a short-term basis, not on a long-term basis. What ends up happening when we are under long-term stress is that we have an elevation of our cholesterol levels. Not only do we have an elevation of our LDL cholesterol (bad cholesterol), but also we have a concurrent reduction in our HDL cholesterol level (good cholesterol).

We have an elevation in our cholesterol levels because we're preparing to do one of two things when we are under stress: we are preparing for a fight or preparing to run away. If you get into a fight, your body, in its infinite wisdom, says, "We need to get some stuff ready to heal you as rapidly as possible." Therefore, the body regulation system raises your cholesterol levels for the healing process. Your body is doing exactly what is right, with the correct substance, when you are under stress. The only problem is that we were not designed to sustain the physiological changes induced by stressful conditions on a chronic (long-term) basis. Unfortunately, in our western society and our culture today, we are required to.

If you take a statin drug (it doesn't matter which one) to lower cholesterol, are you doing anything at all to correct the cause of the elevation of the cholesterol levels? Absolutely not; your stress level is still the same. Your dietary, sleep, and exercise habits, as well as your toxicity levels, are unchanged. You are eating the same things, your exercise level is still near nothing, and your sleep patterns are poor at best. You have done nothing to correct what caused the elevated cholesterol levels in the first place. You're just lowering a number on your blood test, and your medical doctor tells you that you are doing fine. Do you know how many people on statin drugs who have perfect cholesterol levels on paper still die of a heart attack or stroke? The statistics are eye opening.

Clearly, this is not simply a question of your cholesterol level being in the correct range. Certainly, it's going to be in range if you take a statin drug, because that drug is going to artificially alter the cholesterol levels. But that doesn't mean you've fixed the problem. It's just a way to change one of the indices on your blood test.

If we had discovered vitamin D in modern times, we would be more likely to label it as a hormone rather than a vitamin because it's used in virtually every tissue in our body. This is similar to your body's widespread use of omega-3 fatty acids along with many other substances I have already mentioned. Vitamin D is manufactured in our bodies using two things: cholesterol and sunlight. If we artificially lower our cholesterol levels and slather on sunscreen to protect ourselves from the sun, we are eliminating the two components essential in manufacturing vitamin D in our bodies. According to numerous research studies, we are driving down our vitamin D levels to extremely low levels. This specific deficiency of vitamin D has led to increases in the incidences of diabetes, heart disease, stroke, and cancer. The travesty is that this deficiency and the problems that it creates are preventable.

When you look at this picture in light of the philosophy of sufficiency and purity of substances in our body, you will see that this philosophy applies to these two integral components of the health and wellness paradigm as well as many other equally critically components. We want to have sufficient quantities of both cholesterol and vitamin D in our bodies so we can manufacture many other substances required for overall health and wellness. We need to have a sufficiency of all of the substances required to manufacture our sex hormones and stress hormones, as well as vitamin D.

When we take statin drugs to alter our levels of cholesterol rather than dealing with the underlying causes of its apparent excessive levels, we are using external substances/drugs that create secondary problems (side effects) for us. A common one is the muscular pain and joint pain that many individuals experience as a result of taking statins. Statins drive coenzyme Q10 (CoQ10) levels down to the point where they are almost nonexistent. Coenzyme Q10 is a substance that is used in every cell in our bodies to manufacture, or create, energy. If you don't have the adenosine triphosphate (ATP) or the energy source for the muscle cells, they start to break down. Used on a long-term basis, statin drugs can create significant muscular disorders.

The bottom line is that cholesterol is not the bad guy it's been made out to be by the conventional medical system. Cholesterol is in our bodies for good reasons. It's not what's wrong in this equation; rather, it is what we are doing with our current lifestyle choices to create the elevation or alteration in cholesterol levels that is wrong.

SUGAR AND DIABETES

> *"The wise man should consider that health is the greatest of human blessings. Let food be your medicine."*
>
> —HIPPOCRATES

There are different forms of diabetes, but I will be speaking here primarily about adult onset diabetes, the diabetes that most people experience. The number one cause of diabetes is your lifestyle choices. As you are now becoming aware, the flip side to that statement is that the number one cure of diabetes is the alteration of those lifestyle choices. Where does diabetes come from? Why does it occur? The genesis of the problem is in how we treat our bodies.

The components of our diet can be broken down into three primary groups: carbohydrates (which include sugars), fats, and proteins. We also consume a plethora of vitamins and minerals and other cofactors, but foods that fall under one of these three category headings are what we consume on a daily basis. We live in a culture in which we eat food in general, and sugar in particular, in excessive quantities. I actually don't care if you call the carbohydrates that you consume a sugar, a complex carbohydrate, or a simple carbohydrate; ultimately, it's going to be sugar once it gets into your digestive tract and breaks down.

Years ago in the United States, we had what was called the food pyramid. The base was the biggest part, and was composed of carbohydrates. Above that were the proteins, and the fats were at the top. It has since been changed because the US Department of Agriculture didn't know what it should look like any longer. We now have a plate with pie shaped divisions. This is still a very confusing sight for most visitors to the government web site. It also continues to depict the respective components of the "plate" with a grain section about the size of the vegetable section. We have been educated and raised in a society that consumes a grain-based, carbohydrate-laden diet. The problem with this is that carbohydrates, as I said, are converted into sugars rapidly by our bodies. In my practice and in every talk I have ever given, I have asked my patients and individuals in the audience to not make a distinction between sugar and grain-based carbohydrates. I want everyone to consider these types of carbohydrates and sugar as one and the same.

If you don't believe me, take a cracker, put it in your mouth, and chew it for a few seconds. The salivary amylase and other digestive enzymes that are released into your mouth via your saliva will break that substance down into sugar in your mouth, and it will taste sweet to you. We have created a toxicity of sugar and grain-based simple carbohydrates in our western culture. By doing that, we have created a situation where we develop the precursor to diabetes, which is called insulin resistance.

The easiest way to explain insulin resistance is to recognize that you are flooding your bloodstream with sugar. That form of sugar is called glucose in your body, and it is the ultimate food source for every cell in our bodies including those we consider bad cells. Bad cells can take the form of cancer cells, bacteria, yeast, and viruses in our bodies, and they feed on sugar. You can see that by consuming an overabundance of sugar, we are not only inundating the good cells with sugar and causing damage in that way, but also flooding the invaders with the food that they love. The yeast, bacteria, viruses, and cancer cells are gobbling up that sugar, and they proliferate and grow. This level of sugar in our bloodstream is so high that our cells get to a point where they will no longer allow that sugar to be taken into them. They have had enough; they are packed with sugar.

I always use the metaphor of doormen for the cells. The doormen open the cell doors and allow the sugar to go in, and then close the door after the sugar enters. The insulin produced by your pancreas, which is an organ in your abdomen, is released into your bloodstream to bring down your blood glucose levels and allow those doormen to open the doors to let the sugar into the cells.

However, after a certain point, the doormen will lock the doors and not open them anymore because your body has created a state in which the cells no longer respond to the insulin signal and you have developed insulin resistance. What does your pancreas do? Your pancreas says, "Those doormen aren't listening to us. They're not getting the signal, so I guess we'll have to manufacture and send out more insulin to those cells." So the pancreas produces and pumps out even more insulin. But the doormen still refuse to respond to the insulin signal. They continue to say, "Nope, we're still not going to open the doors." Now, you have both high insulin levels and high glucose levels in your bloodstream. That is why the condition is called insulin resistance. You have plenty of insulin, but the cells are resistant to it. You are now in a diabetic mode. Once that sugar stays high for extended periods of time, you have diabetes. There's no place for that sugar to go.

What do we need to do with that sugar? We need to convert it into something else as quickly and as much as possible. What is the body's storage method? Remember there are three things we use as food: carbohydrates and sugars, proteins, and fats. So, the liver says, "Let's start storing this excess sugar," and it stores it anywhere it can by converting it into fat, because your poor liver can't store any more sugar. Your cells are also filled to the brim with sugar. These fat stores are there in case the day should come when you don't have enough food and have to burn that fat as an energy source. Unfortunately, that day never comes, so you get fatter and fatter, and less and less healthy. What do we end up with? We end up with the deposition of fat peri-abdominally, meaning from your knees to your chest. You are going to get a big bottom, big thighs, and a big belly.

Look around you: More and more, we see pear-shaped people who are too fat to slide into a booth at a restaurant and are forced to sit at a table. They also have to pull the chair out so far that they block the aisle. It's unfortunate, but it's happening partially due to ignorance of this process.

So there you have it; adult onset diabetes is an epidemic today because we're loading our systems with sugar and grain-based carbohydrates. Along with that, we are not moving or sleeping right, and we are overstressed.

Remember the Atkins diet? Dr. Atkins said that we should eat more protein, and eliminate sugar and grain-based carbohydrates from our diets. On this diet, patients would eat a protein-based diet for an induction period, generally lasting about two weeks. At that point, the body would go into what was called ketosis, meaning that it was starting to burn up not only fat but also protein. There are a couple of ways in which you can tell when you are in ketosis. One is that you start getting very sweet-smelling breath, almost like an alcoholic would have. You can also use a urine test strip to see if you are in ketosis. Once you reach that point, Dr. Atkins said you can start reintroducing carbohydrates, but from a vegetable-based source (yes, vegetables are carbohydrates and so are fruits). So, if we add in these vegetable-based carbohydrates, we can get ourselves to a balanced point where we are not quite in ketosis, but just teetering on that point. By doing that, you're going to reset your metabolic system so that you are starting to burn up fat as a fuel source.

Your body is very efficient, and it doesn't want to use any more energy than it absolutely has to, so it uses sugar as a primary source of energy. If the body doesn't have a simple sugar to burn, it will move to the next easiest thing that it can use for energy: a carbohydrate, which is a little more complex than simple sugar. These carbohydrates of a grain origin are multiple sugar molecules that are linked together. When the body breaks those bonds, you end up with sugar. But if the body doesn't have access to this next energy source, it then says, "Hmm, okay, what's the next most efficient thing to use?" The next most efficient thing to use is fat.

With the induction period in Dr. Atkins' diet, your body is going to this next level. You are not only burning up fat, but also starting to burn up protein, which is the least efficient fuel source for your body. Your body can break protein into sugar in your body. It can also break carbohydrates into sugars. Your body can break any of these fuel sources into sugar. However, the body wants to make this conversion in the most efficient way possible. So, it starts with sugar, which is the most efficient source of fuel for the body. It doesn't have to expend as much energy to use it. The body in its infinite wisdom then goes to the next most efficient fuel source, which is grain-based carbohydrates. It will then move on to fat as a fuel source. Then, when there is no other alternative, the body will begin the very inefficient process of converting proteins into energy (sugar).

That's the whole philosophy of the Atkins and Paleolithic diets, and it does work to lose weight and reset your metabolism. Unfortunately, many lay people, as well as medical professionals, didn't know the facts about this diet. I know of cases in which people didn't understand that they shouldn't stay on the induction part of the diet for longer than two weeks and stayed on it for a year or more, thus creating significant health problems for themselves. But if you do it appropriately and correctly, you can not only bring down your weight and your blood sugar levels, but reboot your metabolic system so that you are burning things much more efficiently. By eliminating or at least reducing grain-based carbohydrates and supplementing with good quality vegetable-based and fruit-based carbohydrates as opposed to grains, you will create a much more efficient system. This way of eating is much more genetically congruent with the way we were designed to eat.

Dr. Atkins wasn't the first to propose this way of eating or a version of it. I've read studies of individuals in the medical field who did research in the 1920s and 1930s with epileptic patients and had eliminated seizures by putting them on an Atkins-type diet.

We lack the necessary sense of urgency about the need to change the grain-based diet that we consume here in America, and I don't fault the average person because that diet is engrained in the fabric of our culture and society. However, that thinking has to change if we are to survive. The fact is that not only our current disease and sickness care system, but also our culture as a whole, cannot last if we persist in the way we are going. We are going to continue this escalation of the diabetes problem if we don't make changes.

Consider these facts: The current age of onset of adult onset diabetes is no longer actually in the adult years. We are seeing teenagers and young children developing diabetes now. It's coming on earlier and earlier in life because kids are raised on sugar-laden candy, cakes, cookies, and ice cream, along with equally destructive artificial manmade sweeteners. We are simply not consuming real food. It's quite literally a life-threatening situation, and a very slippery slope, which we are rapidly descending.

People have got to wake up. I sound like I'm on the soapbox preaching all the time. It's a simple process when you distill it; we need to eat food, not product.

ALCOHOL AND CAFFEINE CONSUMPTION

> *"It's a great advantage not to drink among hard drinking people."*

> F. SCOTT FITZGERALD,
> *THE GREAT GATSBY*

Today, it is fairly commonplace to read and hear statistics about alcohol's health benefits, but there are also many detriments to alcohol consumption. Let's look at both.

Red wine has been raised nearly to the level of a health food. It has been shown to enhance overall health and wellness because of the benefits of the antioxidant polyphenol compounds it contains, such as resveratrol. This substance is found in the skin of red grapes. However, there have also been numerous research studies that show that the quantity of resveratrol a person would receive from one or two glasses of red wine is not significant. In fact, one would have to consume almost a barrel of wine to get a meaningful concentration of resveratrol in the body's system.

The benefits of alcohol revolve primarily around its blood-thinning capabilities. Part of the reason that people get flushed when they consume alcohol is because it dilates blood vessels, allowing the blood to pass through the vessels more readily. There may also be some additional benefits from alcohol consumption. My grandmother drank a glass of sherry every night before she went to bed and that may have contributed to her longevity. She lived to be 94 years old and was productive that whole time.

According to statistics from the CDC, the percentage of adults 18 years of age and older who consume alcohol on a regular basis is 51.3 percent. If we combine that with infrequent drinkers who consume 1 to 11 drinks in a year, that's 13.6 percent, so really almost 65 percent of our population consumes alcohol. Alcohol-related liver disease caused 15,183 deaths in the past year. Alcohol-induced deaths, which included accidents and homicides, account for 24,518 deaths. We need to factor that negative effect into our overall health and wellness paradigm when we assess alcohol consumption and the use of alcohol as a health-related product.

If you understand that sugar-related diseases and disorders are what we need to prevent and avoid, then you also need to recognize that alcohol is converted to sugar very rapidly and readily in your body by the liver. Therefore, when you consume alcohol you are also increasing your sugar load. According to the CDC, excessive alcohol consumption is the third leading preventable cause of death in the United States. It's associated with multiple adverse health consequences, including the biggie that everyone normally associates with alcohol consumption: cirrhosis of the liver. While I am speaking of cirrhosis of the liver, I want to interject that one of the little known but significant causes of this condition is a new disease that the medical community has added to the list: fatty liver disease. This is not a disease. It is a preventable condition that is caused by the way we lead our daily lives and the lifestyle choices we make. Alcohol consumption is also related to a variety of cancers.

Another interesting piece of information is that alcohol consumption in the Unites States has led the CDC to now list in statistics not only alcohol-attributable deaths, but also "years of potential life lost." When I was looking at the deaths of individuals from alcohol reported in research studies from 2001 to 2004, there were 75,766 alcohol-related or associated deaths. But if you look at the statistics relative to years of potential life lost, the statistics become dire; in the same period of time, there were 2.3 million years of productive life lost, which equates to 30 years of life lost on average for every alcohol-associated death. Potentially you're throwing away 30 years of your life.

When we look at our health and wellness paradigm, we're looking not only at the quality of our lives, but also at the duration of productive life. I noted earlier that our focus must not only be on how long we are going to live, but also on how well and productive we are going to be during the years that we have. My concern about alcohol consumption is that alcohol is a toxic substance or, if you like, a poison in your body. Your liver works very diligently to clean it out as soon as you put it in. This is part of the reason that individuals end up with liver dysfunction as a result of overconsumption or abuse of alcohol.

I always shy away from talking in terms of doing things in moderation, because moderation is a very relative term. You could say, "Yeah, I drink in moderation. I only drink two six-packs a night." We have to look at the negative implications on our overall health and wellness for everything we do, alcohol consumption being one of those things. That said, if you're going to drink, you're better off consuming alcohol that is in some way beneficial to your health. Dry red wine would be an example. Dark beers, which contain sediment of some of the antioxidant constituents of beer, are more beneficial than drinking clarified light beer, which doesn't have the same antioxidant properties.

Recently we have seen a great deal in the media about the dangers of caffeinated energy drinks combined with alcohol. These energy drinks are highly caffeinated beverages and are most often consumed by young people. In a study by Malinauskas et al. 492 college students were surveyed. Of those students consuming caffeinated energy drinks 57% of females and 50% of males combined these drinks with alcohol. These drinks also contain a great deal of sugar and other additives. Look at the negative effects of caffeine on the body. Caffeine can cause headaches, dizziness, abdominal cramps, nausea, vomiting, and even convulsions and tremors. On a short-term basis in concentrated forms, caffeine can cause negative effects to the central nervous system as well as the cardiovascular system. In addition to the insomnia we normally associate with caffeine, it can cause overall excitement, fast heart rate, and increased urination. When we concentrate the caffeine, this magnifies these symptoms and signs.

When we combine caffeine and alcohol, caffeine masks the depressant effects of alcohol. While alcohol is a depressant, causing our systems to slow down, caffeine is a stimulant that does just the opposite, causing our systems to rev up. What occurs when you combine the two in higher concentrations is you will no longer feel the effects of the alcohol in the way you ordinarily would. When you consume alcohol, your reflexes slow or you may slur your speech, which serves as a warning signal to you or those around you that you need to stop or slow down. But when you combine alcohol with high-energy caffeinated drinks the depressant effects are masked, so you will be more likely to consume more alcohol as a result of having the elevated caffeine concentration circulating through our body.

Caffeine does little to speed up the metabolism of the alcohol that you have just consumed, however. Therefore, it doesn't help our livers in any way. Drinkers who consume caffeine and alcohol together are actually three times more likely to binge drink than drinkers who do not use these combined drinks. What's more, individuals who consume alcohol-caffeinated drinks are twice as likely to report being taken advantage of sexually than drinkers who do not use these mixed drinks.

Because of the dangers associated with this category of drinks, I think that state or even federal legislation will ultimately be written to limit or regulate the combination of these two chemicals. When you consider the global use of alcohol and of caffeinated beverages, including coffee, you will find that there are some research studies touting the benefits of both. I believe, however, that the overall negative effect of both substances on our system outweighs the marginal positive effects.

That doesn't mean that you should never consume coffee or alcohol in the health and wellness paradigm. However, you must be judicious in the way you consume these two chemicals. Certainly, the consumption of caffeine in our culture occurs primarily in the form of coffee and caffeinated soft drinks. If you take a look at the effects of caffeine from coffee and the effects of caffeine from tea, they actually affect your system differently. There are numerous research studies touting the benefits of tea to your cardiovascular function due to the antioxidants it contains and its overall enhancement of immune function.

In my practice, I recommend that my patients consume organic green tea as opposed to coffee. When we do our Full System Detox Cleanse Program, which we offer twice a year at our

Center, caffeine consumption is eliminated except for one to two cups of organic green tea per day. One of the significant benefits that patients report back to us is a dramatic change in their sleep patterns as a result of removing caffeine from their diet. They also experience an overall rise in their energy level. Most of you might assume that you would see just the opposite, because you may have been using the caffeine as an energy boost. If you're taking your coffee fix two or three times a day, you are generally stimulated by that fix. Part of the reason you feel that you require that caffeine jolt is because your adrenal glands are fatigued. You are no longer producing a sufficient level of cortisol and other adrenal hormones. These hormones typically cycle at different levels at different periods throughout the day. Instead, you're trying to stimulate your body using caffeine as a replacement for those adrenal hormones. When you remove the caffeine from your diet, you begin cleaning the body out, and you'll start to see a return of your natural rhythms and the natural cycles of your body's clock. Your sleep cycle will become more stabilized and routine, as will other energy cycles throughout your day.

If I were to sum up my thoughts and observations on the use of both caffeine and alcohol without using the term *moderation*, what we need to do is make wise choices regarding these two chemicals. In the past, you may have tended to consume these substances rather thoughtlessly and, like most Americans, on a daily basis. You must always do your best to choose wisely. If you're going to choose an alcoholic beverage, at least choose a dry red wine or a dark beer. If you're going to consume caffeine, do so in the form of green tea as opposed to coffee. I would also encourage you to use an organic form of tea. When we look at the toxicity component of this health and wellness equation, nonorganic tea can be a very heavily herbicide-laden drink.

The use of herbal teas is helpful and beneficial in many ways. There are different forms of herbal teas that are naturally caffeine-free, rather than decaffeinated. If you're looking for a non-caffeinated beverage, an herbal tea may be the right choice for you, and again, you should always choose an organic type if possible.

HOW IMPORTANT ARE FRUITS AND VEGETABLES?

"Prevention is better than cure."

—DESIDERIUS ERASMUS

I discussed carbohydrate consumption earlier and how basing your carbohydrate consumption on grains was dead wrong, despite what the old food pyramid used to encourage. You need to immediately dismiss that old concept and start thinking differently.

First, you need to understand that vegetables and fruits are carbohydrates, and that those foods should be the basis of your diet. You need to change your carbohydrate consumption from a grain-based diet to a vegetable-based diet incorporating some fruits. I emphasize vegetables because they typically have a lower sugar concentration, with a few limited exceptions. They also break down more slowly and uniformly into sugar in your body than grains do for the most part. In my health and wellness paradigm, vegetables and fruits are the key to a healthy diet.

When we look at the choice between conventionally grown as opposed to organic, there are a few things to consider. The terms *natural* and *all natural* are marketing ploys. Natural really means nothing because anything that is grown can be considered natural, because, for example, it may have come from a tree. I recently went into a big natural food chain store looking for some dark chocolate. (I eat the dark chocolate that the rest of the family won't consume; it's 86 percent to 99 percent cocoa. They buy it for Dad as a gift because they know nobody else is going to eat it.) I was looking through the aisle for some good, organic dark chocolate, and I was amazed by how many chocolates were labeled natural. "Natural dark chocolate"—that doesn't mean anything other than perhaps that it is "minimally processed."

I select organic dark chocolate for the same reasons I recommend organic teas: most teas and cocoa we purchase locally are grown outside of this country. Many of the constraints on pesticide use that are enforced here in the United States do not apply in other countries. By at least attempting to consume an organic form, you are getting the benefit that the US Department of Agriculture inspects those products to ensure they conform to their organic guidelines. There is definitely a difference.

When considering which fruits and vegetables to eat, I would like to see you consuming those that are organically grown, not only because of the more nutrient-rich soil they are grown in, but also because of the way in which this class of fruits and vegetables are propagated and harvested.

Recently, I visited an organic farm and saw the techniques they employed for mulching and soil preservation. Fifty years ago, farmers practiced crop rotation to replenish the soil, a practice that has been largely replaced by the use of nitrogen-based chemical fertilizers. But crop rotation is still practiced on organic farms, where soil is enriched solely with humus and other organic forms of fertilizer. My brother farms and has an organic packing house in California. I know from personal observation how stringent the US Department of Agriculture is in its regulations regarding the production of crops on organic soils. It's not something that just anybody can do. It takes years to have soils certified as organic. Even to process food in an organic facility requires a number of certification steps, both initially and yearly. As an example of the strict regulations associated with producing certified organic food, my brother is not permitted to allow a piece of conventionally grown fruit to touch the same packing line on which organic produce is being processed.

Most organic facilities are purely organic. They don't have conventional produce running anywhere near the organic lines because if they do it's too easy to have cross-contamination. If that occurs, the line will be shut down. There are regular inspections of organic facilities to ensure that they're not cross-contaminating.

I've heard a lot of criticism of organic food, and I've seen a lot of research studies on the difference between the nutrient content in organic food as opposed to conventional food. There's no doubt that organically grown food is significantly more nutrient-dense than conventional food. Anyone who questions this should try eating a conventional banana and an organic banana. Try eating a conventional egg and an organically grown and a harvested egg.

You will find that there is a difference in the taste itself. Numerous detailed studies have proven that organic food does contain more nutrients than conventional food,[2] but remember, the key word is *organic*.

I'd like you to start thinking of the term *all natural* as just what it is: a marketing ploy used to sell foods and products. Look for organically produced food when possible, and specifically those that are grown in the United States where the US Food and Drug Administration has inspected and certified them. Certainly, it's difficult to consume a completely organic diet. But if you can, at least incorporate some organic and some locally grown foods; it will be beneficial for your overall health and wellness.

I realize that expense is an issue for many of us in making these choices. Consumption of organic food is generally more expensive. One way to get around that is to buy local. Locally grown fruits and vegetables will not only be tastier, but usually more nutritious. Generally speaking, you can buy organically grown local food for less than non-local food because transportation costs are cut out of the equation.

Our family is very fortunate to have an orchard right down the road from our house; the farmers don't spray as they do at

---

2   E. Palupi, et. al., "Comparison of Nutritional Quality between Conventional and Organic Dairy Products: A Meta-analysis," *Journal of the Science of Food and Agriculture* 92, no. 14 (2012): 2774–2781, doi:10.1002/jsfa.5639; Duncan Hunter et. al., "Evaluation of the Micronutrient Composition of Plant Foods Produced by Organic and Conventional Agricultural Methods," *Critical Reviews in Food Science and Nutrition* 51, no. 6 (2011): 571-82, doi:10.1080/10408391003721701; "Organic Food Is More Nutritious Than Conventional Food," Journal of Applied Nutrition 45 (1993): 35-39, http://www.organicconsumers.org/Organic/organic-study.cfm.

industrial orchards and farms. These farmers still use some of the practices that were used years ago in conventional farming. When you buy local, you're getting foods that are not transported or stored for the length of time that fruits and vegetables are when they are transported across the country or around the world. This is important, particularly when we consider the fact that nutrients diminish in food the longer it has been since harvesting. Thus, the closer to home you can buy fruits and vegetables, the more nutrient-dense they will tend to be.

This will also go a long way toward helping you in reducing toxicities. It will assist you by compensating for deficiencies that you may have acquired, because you are consuming foods that are more nutrient dense. By changing your philosophy on the consumption of carbohydrates from a grain-based diet to a more vegetable- and fruit-based carbohydrate diet, you will make significant strides in improving your overall health and wellness.

OMEGA-3 FATTY ACIDS

"Omega 3 fatty acids are important for normal metabolism."

—WIKIPEDIA

What are some things you can do to enhance your health and wellness? I'd put the consumption of a good, quality omega-3 supplement at the top of the list. You are not likely to get an adequate concentration of omega-3 fatty acids from the foods you eat. You would have to consume a significant amount of wild fish (as opposed to farm-raised fish) or consume a significant quantity of range-fed meat, (lamb or beef) to start nudging your omega-3 fatty acid level up to where it should be. These supplements provide a way for you to increase this nutrient in your body without having to consume these foods and without increasing your expenditures for your weekly grocery purchases enormously.

We have created a situation in which our bodies are toxic in omega-6 fatty acids but deficient in omega-3 fatty acids. We get our omega-3 fatty acids from grasses. We get our omega-6 fatty acids from grains. We consume omega-6 fatty acids not only in the corn and wheat we consume in our antiquated grain-based carbohydrate diet, but also in the pork and beef and farm-raised fish that we consume, which originally had fed on grass and seaweed and algae but now are fed grains. Our omega-3/omega-6 fatty acid ratio is out of balance. We should have about a 1:3 ratio in our bodies. That ratio has become skewed to the point to where we may have a 1:60 ratio.

The problem with omega-6 fatty acids is that they cause inflammation in our bodies, as do grains. Omega-3 fatty acids are anti-inflammatory; they decrease inflammation in our systems, as do vegetables and spices. To reduce inflammation in your body, and by doing so reducing heart disease, cancer, strokes, and diabetes, you must begin incorporating quality omega-3 fatty acids into your diet.

You'll note that I qualified omega-3 fatty acids with the term quality. You have to understand that fish today, and in particular wild-caught fish, is likely to contain myriad toxins, including polychlorinated biphenyls (PCBs) and mercury. Because we're trying to reduce our toxicity, we want the concentration of PCBs and mercury in our omega-3 fatty acid source to be as low as possible. Whether we're adding omega-3s through our food or via supplementation, we need to look at ways to reduce those toxins. If we're using supplements, we need to consider the varieties of fish used to manufacture them, and the purification processes used to extract contaminates or toxins from the fish oils.

The longer a fish lives and the bigger it gets, the more it will bioaccumulate (accumulate a substance in a living organism) toxic substances in its tissues. Substances such as mercury and PCBs are present in the waters in which they live. Therefore, it is wise to extract omega-3 fatty acids from fish that have a shorter life cycle, like sardines or herring. Because they have a shorter lifespan than some of the larger fish like cod that are often used as sources of omega-3 fats, these smaller fish bioaccumulate less of these toxic substances.

According to one study, fish such as grouper, marlin, salmon, sea bass, shark, swordfish, and tuna contain the highest concentrations of mercury. Fish such as cod, halibut, snapper, monkfish, and mahi-mahi contain moderate levels of mercury. Fish that contain the lowest levels of mercury include anchovies, catfish, flounder, sardines, and trout. Quality fish oil supplements are manufactured from smaller fish, like sardines or herring, and have been processed in some way to extract these toxins from the fish oil itself.

The two constituents of omega-3s that are important to your health are eicosapentaenoic acid (EPAs) and docosahexaenoic acid (DHAs). People will go down to the local discount store and purchase their fish oil and never look at the concentration of EPA and DHA. These are the two active, effective elements of omega-3 fatty acids. Even with the supplements, these individuals may not be getting sufficient quantities of these two, key components of fish oil. This is particularly important relative to the use of these omega-3 fatty acids in the prevention and care of a variety of brain disorders, including Alzheimer's and strokes. We have to look at the DHA concentration because that's the form of omega-3 fat that's found in the tissues of the brain. Numerous research studies have shown that consuming a high quality omega-3 fatty acid with a sufficient concentration of DHA will not only reduce the likelihood of stroke, but also reduce the incidence of having a repeat stroke.

You may recall that in 2006 there was a mine collapse in West Virginia. A young man named Randal McCloy was the only survivor rescued from that mine; however, he remained in a coma for several months afterward. His neurologist, Dr. Julian Bailes, had tried everything he could think of to assist this young man in regaining consciousness and recovering from the methane and carbon monoxide poisoning that he had sustained as a result of being trapped in the mine. Not only had Randal sustained damage from these gases to his brain and nervous system, but virtually every other vital organ was beginning to shut down. Randy was at death's door.

For several months, Dr. Bailes was unsuccessful in his attempts to bring Randy out of his vegetative state. Finally, having exhausted every treatment that conventional medicine had to offer, Dr. Bailes boldly decided to try an alternative approach. He prescribed omega-3 fatty acids for Randy, a dose that was about

16 times higher than what is normally recommended. Within a matter of days of receiving these megadoses of omega-3 fatty acids, Randy awoke from his unconscious state and began his recovery. Dr. Bailes attributed the miraculous healing process to his addition of omega-3 fatty acids to this young man's routine medical protocol.

I see dramatic changes in individuals time and time again in my practice with arthritic conditions, skin conditions, and cognitive issues. A variety of maladies respond well to replenishment of deficiencies in omega-3 fatty acids.

One recent study has even demonstrated the positive effects of maternal omega-3 fatty acid levels on infant weight management. In other words, if a mother's omega-3 levels are sufficient during pregnancy, a child's potential to become obese will be reduced. Thus, these health benefits are generational. Mothers who reach and maintain sufficient levels of omega-3 concentration in their own body during pregnancy also provide benefits to their children that are seen later in life.

That's why it's so important to create a sufficiency in your omega-3 levels. This is something that can be checked in a blood test, but is not routinely tested by our standard medical system.

The other essential nutrient that can be tested very easily, but which most medical doctors do not routinely test, is your vitamin D blood level. Every individual who has a blood test on an annual basis should have the vitamin D level tested.

When we consider why you are most likely deficient in these essential nutrients, we must also consider what conventional medicine focuses on today. One of the criteria for bringing drugs to the market is that we must have or must create a problem, so that we can invent a drug to deal with it. The hype from the medical/pharmaceutical industry is all about the evils of cholesterol. I am not saying there is not a problem with the soaring cholesterol levels that are becoming the norm in our western societies. I am concerned, however, with the belief that by driving cholesterol levels down artificially using statin drugs we are actually improving an individual's health. The fact is that by doing nothing to correct what has created the elevation in blood cholesterol levels, we are doing nothing to correct the cause of the problem, which goes back to our lifestyle choices.

A big contributor to our deficiencies in both vitamin D and omega-3, but vitamin D in particular, may be the widespread use of these same statin (cholesterol-lowering) drugs. I spoke earlier about our cholesterol levels and how important cholesterol is in our overall health and wellness. Yet, through the use and even the abuse of statin drugs, many patients are actually creating a deficiency in their cholesterol levels. Once again, I want to reiterate that I am not saying that having high cholesterol does not have adverse health effects; it certainly does. But by artificially reducing high cholesterol levels, we are not necessarily improving our health.

Let's tie this all together with the vitamin D deficiency that is rampant in our society. There's another reason for this widespread problem, and this is an interesting one because it relates to the deficiency in omega-3 fatty acids that most of you suffer from. Omega-3 fatty acids are important to proper skin function, proper cell function, and proper tissue function throughout the body. We have high skin cancer rates today, and those rates are affected by UV radiation exposure. But why are our skin cancer rates so high when our sun exposure rate has been reduced by our largely sedentary, indoor lifestyles and almost fanatical use of sun blocks?

The protective mechanism afforded by sufficient omega-3 fatty acid concentrations in our bodies could be part of this problem, at least relative to the vitamin D deficiency.

These are essential nutrients. The effect of both vitamin D and omega-3 fatty acids on our overall wellness is significant when we look at cancer rates, diabetes, and other conditions. Many of these conditions can be eliminated and the percentage of our population that experiences them reduced significantly just by increasing their omega-3 fatty acid consumption and vitamin D concentration.

Depending on what lab you use, it's going to vary a bit, but the normal healthy range of vitamin D should be from 30 nanograms per milliliter (ng/mL) to 100 ng/mL. If you're at 30 ng/mL, you are still deficient in my book. Your levels of vitamin D are too low. Supplementation with vitamin D at 2,000, 3,000, even 4,000 to 10,000 international units of vitamin D on a daily basis—a level that used to be considered toxic by the conventional medical world—is not excessive in our society today. Certainly you need to monitor your level through routine blood tests, but if you were to take only 1,000 international units of vitamin D, that would not be excessive in most cases.

In a fashion similar to the fortification of salt with iodine, we also began fortifying our milk with vitamin D. That smidgen of vitamin D was added to milk because many in our population were deficient in vitamin D and that fact was becoming apparent to the US Food and Drug Administration and the US Department of Agriculture. They concluded that there had to be a convenient way to get vitamin D into the masses. Once again, they looked for a food source that the general population consumed in large quantities, and this time they chose milk, so they threw some vitamin D in that milk product that was being processed through pasteurization and homogenization. Unfortunately, in this processing, a lot of the good qualities of whole raw milk are destroyed.

Those who have ever drank milk from the bulk tank on a farm know the difference between fresh milk and what you buy in stores. When you drink fresh milk, it tastes like what the cow has eaten. That's why if a cow eats onion grass, the dairy farmer has to get rid of the milk. When milk is processed, vital nutrients are destroyed. For example, probiotic bacteria are killed off and proteins are altered. The infusion of vitamin D into milk is considered a fortification process. The fortifying of processed food invariably involves removing or destroying certain nutrients through the processing production line and then adding some nutrients back in that are thought to be beneficial. But what is added back in are typically synthetic nutrients manufactured from substances that start out very dissimilar to the end product. For instance, we fortify cereal because we've extracted all of the good constituents from the grains to begin with by processing it, so this is an attempt to throw a little nutrition back in that food product.

This really is a very strange process when you think about it. Our nutrients should be coming from our food, not from the synthetic nutrients that we put back into the food product being created, which in fact had many of the nutrients extracted in the first place.

"You are not *what you eat: You are what you digest and absorb!"*

~DR. DOUGLAS G. PFEIFFER

The old adage says, "You are what you eat," but in fact you are what you can digest and absorb. As we age, our digestive processes slow, our stomach acidity and enzyme production reduces, so we end up not digesting our food as well and, therefore, not absorbing nutrients from it. Intestinal linings and permeability change also, and therefore, the ability to absorb nutrients from our food further reduces. Consequently, many of us in our senior years become malnourished (in spite of the fact that we may be eating a relatively correct diet), because our digestive and absorption processes are significantly impaired.

One of the keys to being able to not only digest but also absorb nutrients from our food begins when we put it into our mouth. We need to be able to masticate, or chew, to break down our food as much as possible before we swallow it. Unfortunately, in our high-speed, fast-paced world, we eat too fast. You may not really think about the process of eating. Instead, you're likely to be multitasking while you are eating. Consequently, you are not beginning the digestive process correctly by breaking your food down sufficiently at the onset of eating.

Therefore, the first thing I would recommend is that you chew your food longer and better. Some of you may be compromised in this ability due to poor dental health or the use of dentures. This will impair your ability to break food down. But if you begin to be more conscious about the process of taking the time to chew your food sufficiently when you eat, most of you will find that not only will your digestive process improve, but your health will improve as well. Another part of the digestive process that happens as you chew is the release of salivary enzymes. These enzymes begin to break food down in your mouth if you have it there long enough for this process to occur. Unfortunately, due to a number of factors including dehydration and a lack of proper nutrition, many people don't salivate well enough or produce enough salivary enzymes to begin the process of breaking food down while it is still in the mouth.

I tell my patients to chew their food 30 times before they swallow it. It's torture for most people. When my patients try to eat more mindfully, many of them report to me how hard it was to break the habit of just putting something in their mouth, chomping on it a couple times, and swallowing it. If you really begin to chew your food properly, you will enjoy the food more, and you certainly will allow your body to absorb more of the nourishing substances from the foods that you consume. It will take some getting used to, because it not only takes more time, but tires your jaw muscles. It is important to remember that digestion begins in the mouth, and you've got to give it a good start.

The next phase of digestion after you swallow your food is to ensure that it breaks down correctly in your stomach. Stomach acidity is critical to digestion. The pH, or (in this case) the acid level of your stomach, ranges anywhere from 1.5 to 3.5. This is a very acidic environment; the most acidic area of the entire digestive tract. That pH balance is critical because your stomach is where you will break your food down into its specific components. I see more and more of the secondary effects of reduced stomach acidity particularly in my ageing patients. This problem is worsened by the little-known consequences of the use and abuse of an entire class of drugs that reduce or retard the production of stomach acid. These drugs are used to treat GERD, or gastro-esophageal reflux (what we used to call heart burn). Many of these drugs are designed not only to neutralize stomach acidity, but also to stop the production of essential stomach acid. If you are using these drugs or simply getting older, your ability to break food down in the stomach is going to be significantly compromised.

The other process that occurs during the breakdown of your food is that the stomach, which is a big muscle bag, must contract and start churning the food. Gastric motility, or the ability of the gastrointestinal (GI) tract to contract, hinges on a number of factors. These include not only nerve input from your brain to the stomach, but also your ability to maintain bodily motion. If you exercise regularly, the motility of your digestive tract will increase, and consequently, you'll have a better flow of food through your GI tract.

As we progress in our journey down through the rest of the digestive tract, we come to the next important area in the absorption of nutrients: the small intestine, the largest portion of your digestive tract. This is the area where we absorb most of our nutrients. Again motility, or moving the food bolus through that small intestine, is essential. It's vital that the food does not become static in your small intestine.

The integrity of the lining of the small intestine must be maintained and kept healthy to enhance the absorption of nutrients. The small intestine is about 21 feet long and has what are called villi, little ridges throughout its internal lining that significantly increase the overall surface area. This allows for more of the small intestine to be in contact with your food as it passes through, which in turn allows for more efficient and better overall absorption of nutrients from the food you eat. As you age, these villi start to atrophy. A part of the reason for this breakdown is caused by what you put through your bowel. It is also due to the fact that you don't exercise the bowel, or keep it moving and functional. Again, exercising the entire body will enhance this important function, which is specifically bowel motility.

Feeding improper foodstuffs to the bowel can create a toxic environment inside the bowel. Remember that proper health of the entire GI tract requires the correct maintenance of the acid-base balance in our digestive tract. The stomach should have a pH of about 2.5 and should be the most acidic area of the digestive tract. The small intestine has a much higher pH and, therefore, is less tolerant to acidity. Because so much of the food we eat is grain-based, not only do we create an acidic environment, but also an inflammatory environment in the bowel. Grains are inflammatory to our bodies because they contain high concentrations of inflammatory omega-6 fatty acids.

If you are eating the standard American diet, you are inflaming your body. As you load heavily processed grain-based food products into your bowel, you are creating an inflamed and irritated lining of the GI tract and, in particular, the lower bowel area. This speeds up the breakdown of the digestive tract, and the lining of the digestive tract begins to thin, causing a poorer absorption rate of nutrients through your small intestine. As the lining of the large bowel begins to break down, you will develop a condition called leaky gut syndrome. This condition causes substances to pass through the bowel wall in your intestines that should not normally be allowed. This will kick off a plethora of autoimmune responses, which can create a variety of allergies and toxicities and varied autoimmune responses in areas far from the GI tract. Your body is just doing the best that it can in an attempt to compensate for these invading foreign substances. Thus, you can actually create autoimmune syndromes by producing antibodies against your own body tissue as a result of this condition.

The overall health and wellness of the small and large intestines is critical for proper health. Health of the GI tract is propagated and perpetuated by the use of proper nutrition. You must begin moving toward eating a plant-based diet. This will enhance the overall function of your GI tract.

The large intestine is the area where your body will save water through the process of water reabsorption. The body is designed to conserve water because the body is comprised of about 70 percent water. The large bowel is also a region of the GI tract, which has a great deal of lymphatic tissue associated with it. The lymphatic tissue is the garbage disposal system of your body. It's a component of your immune system. It is immune tissue that protects you from invaders such as bacteria, viruses, and fungi. We have a high concentration of these lymphatic tissues around the bowel and the gut.

There is another component of your immune system that resides in your bowel: probiotic bacteria. There is a symbiotic, or mutually beneficial, relationship that occurs between the good health–producing probiotic bacteria in your small and large intestines and the overall health and wellness of your body, specifically your immune system. Symbiotic in this instance means that there are two partners in this relationship, one being our bodies and the other being the probiotic bacteria that should inhabit our bowel.

The probiotic bacteria are an immune-enhancing component of our body. It should be the first, biggest, and most effective component of our immune systems. Our only contribution to this wonderful relationship is that we have to feed our partners, the beneficial probiotic bacteria. What we should be feeding them is good, healthy fiber because that's what they need to thrive. Unfortunately, once again with our product-based diet, we are not feeding them fiber. We are consistently feeding them sugar. What ends up happening in our system is that a lot of the good probiotic bacteria die off. The imbalance that this creates in our gut can lead to an unhealthy proliferation of specific colonies of the probiotic family, including certain yeasts. We can also host invasive fungi that become prolific and start taking over in that environment. Over the last five to six decades, we have further reduced our probiotic bacteria by consuming excessive quantities of antibiotics, thus compromising our immune systems even more.

Antibiotics were inarguably a godsend after World War II because up until their discovery we had nothing that would kill certain forms of bacteria. Unfortunately, between World War II and the early 2000s, antibiotic therapy was abused and overused in this country where doctors routinely prescribed them for every little infection. Often these infections were viral; antibiotics are ineffective against viral infections.

Fortunately, we're seeing that tide reversed, but it's happening too late to prevent a lot of damage that has already been done to our bodies, our society, and our culture as a result of this abuse. In the birthing process, infants used to receive their initial inoculation of health and immune-producing probiotic bacteria through fecal and vaginal discharge from their mother. Through this initial inoculation, the infant's immune system is kickstarted. Today, we have decimated the good probiotic bacteria in our bowels by abusing antibiotics to the point where the initial inoculation that infants are supposed to receive from their mothers during the birth process is no longer occurring.

There are other immune-enhancing aspects of not only the birth process, but also particularly the initial nursing process, and I strongly recommend that every new mother begin by nursing her newborn so her child receives at least the initial colostrum, the highly immune-beneficial milk from the mother that's produced in the breasts, immediately after childbirth. Formula-fed infants are certainly not receiving this initial inoculation, and they are not benefitting from the stress-relieving, esteem-building aspects that both mother and child receive through the process of nursing. Consequently, the immune systems of most infants being born today are being compromised from birth.

What I want you to understand from this explanation is that the birth process today is not as it was intended to be. Our current lifestyles have disrupted the balance in the relationship between the good probiotic bacteria that we should house in our bowel and the overall immune system's ability to function to protect our bodies.

What can you do to support this health-producing, natural symbiotic relationship between your body and the probiotic bacteria that your bowel should house? Start by consuming a high-quality, broad-spectrum probiotic supplement. This supplement should contain the numerous probiotic bacteria that should be normal inhabitants of your bowel. Taking these supplements will re-inoculate your bowel and enhance your overall immune function. Also, start feeding those probiotic bacteria in your bowel the correct food: plant-based, high-fiber foods. These foods are referred to as prebiotics. By doing those two things, you can reestablish probiotic growth and a healthier immune system, which will enhance your overall longevity as well as your health and wellness.

That acidity varies throughout the bowel, but it is often compromised not only by the foods you eat, but also by the drugs you consume. Many drugs are acidic, and that acidity contributes to the overall acid levels in your body. Likewise, a lot of the foods that we eat are acidic and inflammatory and contribute to the overall decimation of that acid-base balance in your body.

To balance the acidity and alkalinity in your body, you need to be aware of the relative alkalinity and acidity of the foods you eat. The traditional American grain-based diet, which is comprised of refined breads, pasta, and cereals, is made up of bad carbohydrates. These are foods that you likely grew up with and are accustomed to, but in fact these are foods that we've adopted in our culture relatively recently. The overconsumption of these foods in our standard American diet is primarily due to cultural, societal, and marketing pressures. When I say this to patients, I hear responses like, "Breads have been eaten since ancient times, and pasta is part of the Mediterranean diet that we hear so much about. I thought that was supposed to be healthy. How can those things be bad for me?"

Let's explore that question a little. As a species, we have been consuming these foods for thousands of years, but the bread you eat today, when compared to that eaten in earlier eras, would have been considered cake back then. I say this primarily due to the fact the flour that we use today is so "ultra refined" compared to what was consumed hundreds of years ago. To individuals of that era it would have had the texture and consistency of what they would have considered to be cake. Breads that were consumed in an earlier era were made from grain milled with stone, which in itself contributed minerals to the flour. Remember, though, the entire grain used then is unlike the grain used today. Today, the bran is usually removed from the grain when the grain is refined to form flour. Unfortunately, the extracted bran contains a plethora of valuable nutrients. The breads that were consumed years ago contained a healthy amount of fiber. Many of the grain-based breads that we eat today have had the fiber removed to a great extent, but then the processors try to put some of the nutrients and fiber back in to this manufactured food product so that they can then market it as a high-fiber bread, cereal, or pasta.

Another reason to avoid these highly refined food products is because these types of grain-based carbohydrates are broken down into sugar very rapidly in our digestive tracts. A vegetable and low glycemic fruit-based carbohydrate diet will lead to a more balanced blood sugar level because these types of carbs are broken down more slowly. Some fruits, however, contain relatively high sugar content. These are higher glycemic fruits. The primary type of sugar that you receive in fruits is fructose. This is a different type of sugar than what you produce when the grains that you consume are broken down. Even though you believe that you are going to be healthier because you are eating a lot of fruit, it is critical to remember that you can still be receiving a high quantity of sugar from many fruits.

Many people feel that consuming a smoothie is healthy. For some individuals, juicing or making a drink in your blender that contains mostly green leafy vegetables can be beneficial to their overall health and wellness. However, in my experience, most people's smoothies are mostly made up of high-glycemic fruits, so that they are getting a fairly high sugar load in each gulp. You can easily become diabetic by consuming too much fruit just as you can from consuming too many grain-based foods. Consequently, for you to begin the process of driving your overall health and wellness in the right direction, increase your vegetable intake more than your fruit intake.

In changing your diet, I recommend that you use a step, or tiered, process. When I begin the process of getting my patients off grains, we gradually transition them. Educating them to understand that vegetables are where they are going to get the better form of carbohydrates is the first step. This alone will be hugely beneficial to the body, to the sugar levels, and to the inflammation in the body. I may have my patients begin a full system detoxification cleanse in my office to assist in "cleaning house." When we begin cleaning their systems, by getting rid of a lot of the toxic chemicals and other substances that have been stored in their bodies, they will begin to feel the difference. The really redeeming part of the process for patients is when others begin to notice the change in them. One of the places that the body will store toxic substances is in the fat cells of the body. The body can't always excrete these substances because it may already be overloaded with toxins, so it has nowhere else to put the garbage.

The body is amazing, particularly in its wisdom in managing its chemistry. To rid itself of waste, it uses the methods of excretion, which we normally think of as occurring through our bowel or urine. But the body will also use your breath and skin to get rid of toxins. Often, I find patients who have toxic overloads who present with skin irritation. I've treated patients who have been diagnosed with psoriasis, for example, and by simply cleaning up their diets and adding some nutritional supplements in which they may be deficient, the psoriasis resolves. It's important to know that many skin conditions that result in skin irritations may be due to a toxicity the body is having difficulty eliminating. Therefore, toxicities and any concurrent deficiencies must be considered and evaluated in such cases.

If the body can't get rid of a toxin, it will often store the substance in fat. We frequently see a patient go through our process of detoxification and lose weight because this process requires a dramatic change in the way most people eat. As they lose weight, they burn fat. As they burn fat, they release toxins into their system. This is why I call our program a detoxification program, or a full system detox cleanse. As they release these toxins, it's vital that the portals are open so they can get these toxic substances out of their body. We want to push toxins through the bowel as much as possible. The other main method used to excrete toxins from the body is urine. If these two portals are not allowing for excretion, or the toxic load is greater than the ability of the body to use these two pathways, then the breath and skin may be used.

Many of you have seen how these pathways are used when you get extremely ill. Consider how your urine color changes, how the smell of your urine changes, and how the look, texture, and odor of your stool changes. It may become very soft or loose. Sometimes the stool may become dark or the odor may be very foul. That's because your body is getting rid of toxins. In that case, it may be bacteria, viruses, or another bioload coming through your bowel and urine. When individuals go through a detoxification process, I want to ensure that the excretion of these substances take place concurrently with the expulsion of the toxic elements from the tissues and cells.

Another component of your health and wellness paradigm that I'd like to see everyone do is to begin the process of controlling the quantity of food consumed. The quality of your food is very important, but quantity is no less important. Numerous research studies have shown that by consuming fewer calories you can significantly increase your longevity. One study referenced the fact that by reducing your intake of food by 1/3, you will increase your longevity by 20 percent.

How do you accomplish this? How can you create a portion control system? One of the main reasons that we eat so much is because food is so plentiful in this country. For most of us, we don't have to worry about food being available. When they were hungry, my kids used to complain that they were starving. I gave the same response every time, "You are not starving. You don't know what it means to be starving. You are simply hungry." It is important not only for our kids, but also for each one of us to realize that the word *starving* should be reserved for specific and all too prevalent situations in our world, and not applied to a delayed meal. When a meal is delayed, don't let your hunger run away with you; eat until your body is satisfied, but not full.

What do you do when you're hungry? If you're like most people, you simply run to the vending machine, throw a buck in, and pull out a candy bar or some other product. It's not really your fault; you've been educated to think that's what you're supposed to do. A recent candy manufacturer's marketing campaign on television suggested that when you eat their candy bar, it changes your personality! In fact, what is really occurring is that you have allowed your blood sugar to reach a significantly low level. You may even be on your way to becoming hypoglycemic. Then, when you jam a sugar-laden food product into your mouth, you spike your blood sugar level. By spiking and dropping your blood sugar levels over and over again, you are creating a prediabetic/diabetic lifestyle.

When we talk about reducing the quantity of food you're eating, that doesn't mean you need to reduce the frequency in which you consume food. One of the simplest ways that you can create this reduction in consumption is to reduce the size of your plate. It's so simple that it almost sounds ridiculous, but it works. If you use a smaller plate, you take less food, and you will eat less. Eat a smaller portion of food and then have a snack later in between meals. Unlike some species, we are genetically designed to graze, not to gorge ourselves. Certain carnivores—wild dogs, for instance—are designed to gorge themselves when food is available, then not eat for an extended period of time, presumably because they have to make the most of what they have killed that day. We, as a species, are omnivores. We eat a variety of foods including vegetables, fruits, and meat. We are designed to consume less food at a time and, therefore, to eat more frequently.

Most people today don't eat breakfast, in spite of the fact that breakfast is the most important meal of the day. It's breaking your fast. You have been sleeping for (hopefully) about eight hours, and your body has used its food reserves. Even though it's been in a subconscious reduced metabolic state, your body is going to need something to get it going again. It needs to replenish blood sugar levels. Breakfast is a critical meal. I drive past a donut shop in the morning on my way into my office, and I typically see people lined up to get their sugar fix. They're loading up on refined carbohydrates/sugars. The grain-based carbohydrates that they are consuming have sugar added in high quantity. They will add to that a coffee with more added sugar, or worse yet, a latte, artificially stimulating their bodies and forcibly waking them up with caffeine and sugar. This is typically necessary because they did not receive a restful sleep the night before. That's their extremely unhealthy start for their day.

How do they feel about an hour or two from then? They feel fatigued, tired, and sluggish, so what do they do? They have more coffee in an attempt to compensate for the adrenal fatigue that they have created and are perpetuating every day through this same process. This goes on throughout the days, weeks, and years as their bodies slowly and progressively deteriorate. Oftentimes, these individuals contribute further to the problem by skipping lunch. Then what do they do? They consume a large carbohydrate-laden dinner, which may consist of a large plate of pasta or piles of french fries. Consequently, they create a rollercoaster ride in their blood sugar levels often to the point where their normal physiological responses are compromised. In other words, they're pumping out insulin after they've taken a big sugar load first thing in the morning, which opens up the doors to those cells and packs them with as much sugar as can fit into the cells.

What happens with the rest of that excessive sugar load? It is stored in the liver as glucagon to be used later. Your body will also store that sugar as fat.

Once your body has shoved all of that excess sugar into the cells, and the cells have stored what they can, your sugar level plummets. Now you don't have enough sugar circulating in your blood stream. With that sudden drop in your blood sugar level, you've got to re-juice it again. This is what occurs as you are creating a hyper-/hypoglycemic condition of prediabetes. You are simply preparing to become a full-fledged diabetic.

By controlling your portions of good-quality, low-glycemic foods (food that will be converted into sugar in your system more gradually), you will enhance not only your longevity, but also your function on a daily, even hourly, basis. You'll have more energy, you won't need to jolt your system with caffeine and sugar, and you will live a longer, healthier life.

This is a simple process. You begin the process by exercising portion control at breakfast and eating a little snack about ten o'clock. This could consist of a handful of almonds or an apple. You should then eat a portion-controlled meal at lunch, and then have another little snack in the afternoon. You eat a portion-controlled dinner, and then perhaps a small snack in the evening about seven or eight o'clock. Eating this way will help you not only lose weight, but you will also feel much more energy and stamina. In other words, you will become healthier. You will have a more balanced blood sugar level throughout the day, and as a result, the potential for you to develop diabetes will be significantly reduced.

I have a patient who consulted me originally because her blood sugar level was 310. She originally had a Glycohemaglobin A1C reading (a long-term [two to three month] measurement of your blood sugar) of 13.1. To put this in perspective, the fasting glucose level should be under one hundred. Your A1C should be in the range of five to eight. She had lost a great deal of weight about two years prior. She stated in our initial meeting that she was eating well. When I asked her what she was consuming, she stated that she was eating whole grains, breads, and pastas. These are all the wrong things. This used to be the way that diabetics were taught to eat, but we know now it's wrong.

What she—and you—needed to do was to eat frequent meals, specifically of a low-glycemic, plant-based diet with some meat. That's our genetic programming; in Paleolithic times, that's the way our ancestors ate. We were a hunter-gatherer race. We were designed to eat what we could forage, kill, pick from a vine or tree, or dig out of the ground. The further we get from that, the less healthy we'll be.

LIFESTYLE CHOICES

> *"Take care of your body. It's the only place you have to live."*

~JIM ROHN

What are the costs of eating right? Eating the way I have been describing to you is not necessarily more expensive, provided you do it correctly. You have to use good shopping sense when eating a healthy diet.

Most people think that they have to eat only certified organic food, which would be prohibitively expensive. That simply is not the case. You can buy locally grown vegetables at a farmer's market; you do not have to go to posh grocery stores. You don't have to spend a lot of money to eat a healthy diet.

You do have to be willing to redirect some of your budget toward foods that are going to be beneficial for your body, instead of using those same dollars on things that are not beneficial. Look at our homes, for instance. How many homes do you see that don't have a satellite dish on their roof? We've got to get our priorities straight. We've got to understand that living a productive, healthy, and healthful life is what our goal must be.

Inevitably, even when you've made the leap to eating correctly, you're bound to encounter situations in which you will have limited choices. You may be at a picnic or at a friend's house where they have prepared foods that are not ideal for your new eating habits. When you find yourself in these situations, and you will, you will need to make the best choices that you can. I have been there; I have had to eat salad or scrape the toppings off of a pizza and eat them and not the dough. It may require some creative on-the-spot thinking, but it's doable when you realize how important these choices are to your overall health and wellness.

We are undoubtedly in a health care crisis in this country. You need to step up and take responsibility for your own health. So decide right now: What are you going to do? What changes are you going to make today? What are you going to cut out? How can you solve this dilemma on a personal level right now?

Good health is the best health insurance there is. Doing things to create health and wellness in your body is miles above any marvelous health insurance plan that the government or your employer will provide. The goal is for you to not need to use your health insurance plans, except for emergency medicine.

I don't want you to have to pay for the drugs that are prescribed for conditions that shouldn't exist. I don't want you to suffer from those secondary complications that develop from preventable conditions, such as diabetes. If you practice the four pillars of health that I am teaching you, redirect your thought process, and, if necessary, redirect some of your finances, then becoming healthier is a no-brainer.

It is not necessary to significantly increase expenditures to eat healthy. You just have to be willing to trade an old habit for a new one. Take breakfast, for instance. You may be in the habit of consuming sugared cereals, which are both expensive and unhealthy. Try instead to have some organic plain yogurt, add some strawberries to it, and give it a little crunch with some pecan granola. We call that Dr. Pfeiffer's Parfait at the Center. It's delicious, it's satisfying, and it's great for you. Now, seriously, how hard was that? You simply have to rethink what you're putting into your body. Having said that, understand too that as you go through this transitional process your taste buds and your sense of smell have become accustomed to certain scents and flavors. These particular scents and flavors are for products that you have consumed. Most, if not all, of those products really aren't good for you, but in your past way of thinking, they were yummy.

I've been through this transition. I understand what you're going through as you progress along the road to health and wellness. When you first start this process, eating a salad dressed simply with some oil and vinegar on it or even just vinegar (what I call a "nearly naked salad") may sound like a horrific thought. I see people at restaurant salad bars typically smothering good, healthy leafy green vegetables, peppers, and cucumbers with a product they call salad dressing, and usually there's more of that on their plates than there is vegetables. It's like eating a salad with an ice cream sundae on top to make it palatable.

In my opinion, using salad dressing would be fine at the start of making the transition to health and wellness. At least you're getting some healthy vegetables in your diet. That said, you'll need to start transitioning your tastes away from the salad dressing and learn to love the salad, because the health benefits of the vegetables are seriously undercut by the saturated fats, trans fats, salt, and sugar in that cup of thousand island dressing. Make a gradual transition to some whole, raw foods, and then get rid of the bad stuff like the condiments and dressings that you are using to cover up the taste of the food.

Consider the humble beet: who in the world would eat beets? When you recognize how beets cleanse your liver and gallbladder and how they change your digestive tract, you will make a cognitive change in your thinking and reap these benefits. When I see patients who have constipation, I tell them to buy three beets, boil them, and eat those beats over the next two days. I can practically guarantee that they will have consistent, regular, and full bowel movements.

Yes, buying and eating quality, healthy food requires an investment, both in terms of money and in mindfulness. It's an investment in you. It's an investment in your health. It's an investment in your longevity, and it's an investment in your children and your grandchildren. In Dr. Pottinger's study of cats that were fed appropriate and inappropriate diets, he was able to demonstrate that the cats' degradation was generational. The generations of offspring degraded further and further with every successive generation. This is exactly what we are doing to ourselves. We are creating offspring that are less healthy than we are, and, just as with Pottinger's cats, there comes a point when we will no longer be able to reverse the downward spiraling trend of disease and sickness. That's a terrible thing to do to ourselves and to those we love.

If you're thinking that somehow you're not worth the investment of time, money, or effort it takes to transition to a healthier lifestyle, think again. I can guarantee that you're worth the investment. But if that is not enough for you, then just consider those you love. Aren't they worth your effort? By eating product, and eating incorrectly, we are up-regulating, or turning on, certain genes. Those are often bad genes, like those that create cancer or Alzheimer's. However, by eating correctly, you can down-regulate or turn off those very same genes. Yes, by turning them off, and turning on the good genes, like those that control your immune system or inflammation in your body, you can significantly improve your overall health and wellness.

Do something; take the first step. The first step is expanding your mind to change your belief system to accept that what you're reading is the truth. I will tell you unequivocally that the concepts I am teaching will produce progressive changes in your physiology, but first you must do one thing: You must change your belief system and recognize that you can take charge of your health and not surrender it to someone else. By being a part of the process of creating change in your body, in your physiological system, and in your lifestyle choices, you have taken the first critical step. The rest of it is easy.

By recognizing these truths and taking some simple first baby steps of application, you will see the transition, and I mean see it when you look in the mirror. Other people will say to you, "What are you doing? Something is different about you." I call it "the healthy glow" because people cannot put their finger on it. It's not quantifiable. It's a change. People feel it, see it, and recognize it, but they can't explain it. Friends and family will say, "What are you doing? Something about you is different."

That one change or that one little thing in your life you choose to do differently could be drinking more water. Drink an extra glass of water every day. I don't care if it's just tap water. We don't have to get into all of the special waters and the billions of dollars that people spend every year on water. *Just do something.* When you do that one thing you will find that your body will change. Be open and aware of the change, recognize it, accept it, and then make another change. As you do that and continue to progressively change and improve what you're doing, over time your body will go through a metamorphosis and you will begin to heal from the inside out. The healing capabilities of your body are infinite. Your body can come back from virtually anything.

As we talk in the next section about stress and how it affects your body, you will be amazed at the physiological changes that occur in your body and the physical changes you can see that occur in your body as a result of diminishing your stress. You will see these physiological changes by making these corrective, adaptive changes in your diets and lifestyle that will enhance not only who you are but also how you think about true health and wellness.

CHAPTER 4

THINK RIGHT

"To keep the body in good health is a duty, otherwise we shall not be able to keep our mind strong and clear."

—BUDDHA

Here's an amazing component of the whole health care dilemma we're in: 80 percent of the disorders or diseases for which patients seek care are directly related to stress. As we get into this subject, you'll recognize how many things that we are treating with drugs on a routine basis that are directly related to the stress response.

THE PROBLEM WITH STRESS

We cannot separate the mind and the body when it comes to stress; they work as a functional unit to overcome stressors. Let's first examine the definition of stress: "Stress is a physical, mental, or emotional factor that causes bodily or mental tension." We are all subjected to many stressors every single day. Those stressors can be either positive or negative. Yes, I said positive stressors; not all stress is negative. The physiological stress response, or the body's response to stress, is actually the body's adaptation to any physical, mental, or emotional demand made on your system. Most of us relate stress to the mental or emotional demands placed on us, but these demands can also be physical. Whatever the stressor is, it can only be met by two basic reactions, both of which worked quite well to keep our Paleolithic ancestors alive: stand and fight or run away. When the stressful situation occurs, which our genetics interpret as an attack or assault, we are programmed to do one or the other action.

After one patient went through my stress seminar, "Stress and How It's Killing You," she said, "I really think there's another response that we have besides fight or flight." She went on to say that she thinks that the third response is to float. She meant that we adapt or change physiologically in response to the stressor. In a way, many of us do float in that adaptive phase for extended periods. We don't deal directly with the stressor as we were genetically designed to do. Instead, we just kind of float and let things happen around us. Sometimes, that's the best choice we have for dealing with a stressor when we know there's no way to eliminate the stressor itself. For instance, the stressor may be your boss or even your spouse. Certainly, we may have the option to change things, but due to other pressures, whether family or financial, we may not feel that we're in a position to do so, so we just float.

If we do choose to float, and many of us do, we can create more problems physically and physiologically, because that's not the way we were designed to deal with stress. We were designed genetically to avoid the stressor (run away) or deal with it (fight it) and be done with the stressor. The stressor was meant to be short-term, not long-term chronic stress, which is what we are confronted with today. The fight-or-flight response is a much healthier way to move through the stress. Floating can often lead to more stress, more adaptive physiological change, and ill health.

As we examine the effects of stress, we need to remember how important it is for us to keep things in perspective. One piece of advice I often share with my patients is, "If you want to feel rich, count all the things that you have that money can't buy." Unfortunately, we get sucked into the rat race of comparing ourselves to others. We get into our materialistic world and forget about all of those things that we have to be thankful for. As a functioning individual and someone who wants to be as healthy as possible, you need to take time every morning to remember what you have to be thankful for. Make sure that when you do this you don't forget those little things that we tend to take for granted every day—for example, your eyesight, or the fact that you have both of your arms and legs to support you and thus the ability to walk or run. The daily practice of conscious gratitude helps us to stay balanced and to keep that healthy perspective foremost in our lives.

Dr. Hans Selye is considered the "father" of stress research and has written numerous books on the subject, including one titled *Stress Without Distress*. He describes stress as taking two forms. He calls one form *distress*, which he states is always a disagreeable form of stress. That's the type of stressor that we think of in our day-to-day experiences, the bad stress, if you will. The other form of stress, which he calls eustress, is a pleasant form of stress. This form of stress may be a little more difficult to conceptualize. The best and most familiar example of this form of stress might be the feeling you have on a first date. Remember those butterflies that you felt in your stomach? Those butterflies were a stress response to a positive stressor. This is a good stress. Another example of eustress would be a child anticipating Christmas or a birthday. When you feel like you're so excited that you can hardly sleep, that is an example of eustress. We don't commonly incorporate good stress into our thought process about stress. Another thing that you need to know is that there will only be one time when you have no stress in your life: when you die.

You have stress when you're fully relaxed, and even when you sleep. That is why you dream and have different dream experiences while you're asleep. As many know, a lack of sleep can be a result of stressors that you cannot come to grips with. Let's look at how these stressors affect us and the physiologic changes that occur in our bodies as a result of these stressors.

We are genetically designed to deal well with most stressors on a short-term basis. Most of the stressors that humans experienced in Paleolithic times were short term. We would do one of two things: run away or fight the thing that was stressing (attacking/scaring) us. However, some of those techniques for dealing with the stressor may no longer be culturally acceptable. Today, we are often dealing with multiple stressors on a long-term, or chronic, basis. For example, if you have an occupation that you dislike or, worse yet, you are living with a significant other whom you dislike or you have an issue with, sometimes it's not so easy to disengage from that situation. If your boss is challenging and creating a lot of stress, you cannot just pop him one or run away. You have to deal with that stressor. You have to be exposed to that stressor on a chronic, long-term basis. The adaptive changes that your body goes through with an initial acute stressor are designed perfectly to accomplish their purpose; that is to keep you alive. However, when you are exposed to those very same stressors on a long-term basis, those same physiological changes now become negative and will actually create a variety of conditions that we now label as a disease.

What are these changes, and how do they occur? In response to the stressors to which you are exposed, you will develop an adaptive physiological change. In other words, your body adapts to the stressor without you having to make a conscience effort to do so. Let's look at what happens in a stress response, without any thought on your part: You have an increase in your heart rate and blood pressure. You exhibit a decrease in sex gland function and sex drive. Digestion is shut down. Growth hormone production and cellular immunity are suppressed. Your adrenal glands are stimulated to produce substances that heighten your awareness and all of the other physiological changes such as increased heart rate and blood pressure. Stressors also cause areas of the brain that process emotion and anxiety to be heightened.

The adrenal, or stress, hormones include cortisol and adrenaline. We've all heard about adrenaline. You may feel an adrenaline rush when you're stressed or scared. It causes you to become very aware. Cortisol causes a number of things to occur in your body on a long-term basis, and one of those things is the deposition of fat. You will have increased fat being deposited in your body when you have heightened cortisol levels. As a result of these hormonal changes, you will also have an increase in your heart rate and blood pressure. Your blood vessels will also constrict. Your blood cholesterol will also increase; LDL cholesterol, the so-called bad cholesterol, goes up and HDL cholesterol, the so-called good cholesterol, goes down. LDL cholesterol is used in wound healing. In response to what it perceives as a physical threat, your body is preparing itself to heal a potential wound, in case you have to fight your attacker. This is a pretty wonderful system of adaptation that we have been blessed with, but it is not so great when that stressor becomes long term.

When you are under stress, your sensitivity, or consciousness of your environment, shoots up. You become more alert physically, mentally, and emotionally. You feel things more acutely. This can be a very negative effect when it occurs on a long-term basis. If you have an increased sensitivity, you have an increased pain level. If you are already experiencing pain, for instance, from inflammation in your body, then that pain will be heightened as a result of a chronic, long-standing stressor.

You experience an increase in clotting factors in your blood as a result of an acute stressor on a long-term basis. You will also experience an unfortunate loss of bone density as a result of chronic stress because your body will pull calcium out of bone and begin to circulate it in the blood stream so that it can be used at the site of an injury to heal more rapidly. On a short-term basis, this is a wonderful way for the body to prepare to heal an injury; however, on a long-term basis, this is a way to create another one of the diseases of our modern society, specifically osteoporosis. We also experience a breakdown of muscle tissue and connective tissue under the physiological effects of long-term stress. These are all physical and physiological changes that occur as a direct response to a chronic stressor.

Now, let's look at some of the cognitive changes and hormonal changes that occur as a direct response to a stressor. Under stress, you will experience a concurrent decrease in short-term memory, your ability to concentrate, and cellular immunity. We also will see a decrease in the hormone serotonin, a hormone that's required to assist you with sleep. Psychological conditions such as depression and anxiety can be initiated or magnified by chronic stress. Chronic stress causes a reduction in both growth and sex hormone levels as well. You will begin to develop a resistance to insulin with exposure to a chronic, long-term stress.

When we examined blood sugar, we learned that when there's too much blood sugar in your blood stream you develop an insulin resistance. When you are living with chronic, long-term stress, your body is doing the right thing. It's trying to get you ready to either run, or to heal yourself in case you sustain an injury when you fight. You will obviously need extra fuel to deal with either one of the outcomes of your short-term stress, whether you stand and fight or run. In accordance with that need, your body is trying to increase your supply of energy, which for the body is derived from sugar. So to meet this need, the body begins increasing your blood sugar levels. When this happens on a long-term basis, you will begin to create insulin resistance and ultimately develop diabetes.

Because you also experience increased feelings of stress, on a long-term basis, your stressor will create more psychological stress for you. Increased fear, increased anxiety, and increased depression are the result. Brain centers for instinctual behavior become stimulated. This means that areas of factual learning and focus shut down. You don't need to be able to memorize the Gettysburg Address when you're under stress; you need to run or fight, so you're not going to have a good learning capability when you're under chronic stress. You can see how this affects students in college or anyone who's in a new job. Attempting to adapt to a new job can be challenging enough because of the stress that you experience due to this change in your life and routine. Adding to those stressors is the fact that now, when you really need to be able to learn a number of new things quickly in your new job, your short-term memory is inhibited by your stress.

There are many accounts of individuals who have been in extremely stressful situations—for example, police officers in a gun fight—who relate after the event is over that they experienced mental tunnel vision as the situation was occurring[3]. They see and hear nothing around them except what they are focused on: the bad guy and the possibility of being wounded or killed. The areas of the brain that we would expect to be heightened are actually dampened. Once that short-term stressor is relieved—when the bad guy runs away or surrenders—then these brain activities are turned on again. There are accounts of individuals who have shot and killed someone in the line of duty and they could not hear their own gun shots. They could not hear the shell casing hit the ground or anyone screaming or yelling. Immediately afterward, those hearing sensations were turned on and they heard every-thing around them clearly once more. They had little or no

---

3   Steve Drzewiecki, "Survival Stress in Law Enforcement," (An applied research
    project submitted to the Department of Interdisciplinary Technology as part of the
    School of Police Staff and Command Program, Traverse City Police Department,
    September 20, 2002).

knowledge of the incident other than what they had their tunnel vision focused on. This extreme state is designed to allow you for a short duration to be so acutely focused that you can direct all of your mental and physical energy on the assailant/stressor and eliminate that stressor.

Short-term memory is reduced when we are under stress. When that stressor continues long term, you can see how it can lead to the signs and symptoms that we associate with early dementia. There are many studies that indicate that chronic stress will cause the onset of dementia or Alzheimer's. There are also studies that have proven that the brain shrinks in size and dimension when an individual is exposed to chronic, long-term stressors.

Your body heightens instinctual behavior during a stressor. In your mind, you create an imprint of how you will react to that stressor the next time it occurs, and that imprinted reaction occurs the next time without you even thinking about it. When the saber tooth tiger attacks the first time, you may have to think a little bit about what you're going to do. The next time it happens, you don't think, you just do. You have preprogrammed your brain at that point to instinctively know what to do. This is why the body will shut down short-term memory. This is why it also shuts off the factual learning centers during these periods of extreme stress. All of these changes in your physiology occur for one purpose, your survival, so that you will live and learn what to do the next time that particular stressor occurs. The way the system is designed to deal with stress is absolutely perfect on a short-term basis.

The hormones of increased sensitivity begin going into increased production mode when you are under stress. You have two divisions of sensitivity. One of the divisions is sensory: touch, taste, smell, sight, and hearing. These centers will be heightened when you are under stress. If you have already been experiencing chronic pain from an ankle injury, when you are concurrently under chronic, long-term stress you will experience increased pain from your ankle injury. The pain will be heightened, so instead of the scale of pain being a two or a three, it's now an eight or a ten. This plays into many conditions that people are diagnosed with today, such as fibromyalgia syndrome, chronic fatigue syndrome, or any other long-standing chronic pain issue.

Let's say you have chronic neck pain. If you're in a job or a relationship that is extremely stressful, that neck pain is going to be worse as a result of the chronic stress to which you are subjected on a daily basis. This pain syndrome may even build to the point of being disabling. We often relate heart disease and heart attacks to chronic stress, but cancer can be directly related to chronic stress. Remember, our body's immune system is dampened as a result of stress. When that stress continues over a long period of time, your immune system is suppressed. When you factor in our daily exposure to cancer-inducing cell mutations, the connection to increased incidence of cancer as a result of stress makes sense. When your immune system is functioning properly, cancer cells are killed off by your own immune system. If, however, your immune system is suppressed due to chronic stress, the cancer can take hold and overwhelm your system.

A complicating factor to all of the good changes that you may make in your diet is that if you're under chronic stress your sugar level will go up in your bloodstream as a direct result of the chronic stress. There's nothing that taking a drug to lower your sugar level will do to correct the cause of your high blood sugar levels because stress itself is the cause.

These diseases of our modern society are actually diseases of adaptation. Conditions such as diabetes, hypertension, heart disease, and cancer go well beyond the simple headache that we would normally relate to the stress in our lives. If we look at the list of conditions that are directly related and attributable to chronic stress, we can include obesity, depression, anxiety, fatigue, chronic pain, osteoporosis, fibromyalgia, sleep disorders, decreased sex drive, erectile dysfunction, decreased fertility, accelerated aging, Alzheimer's, attention deficit disorder (ADD), and attention deficit hyperactivity disorder (ADHD). The direct cause of weight gain is related to increased cortisol levels. Cortisol is an adrenal hormone that our bodies produce as a direct result of stress. This hormone will indirectly cause other diseases and disorders to occur. If we really extrapolate, we can also include cancers of the colon, kidney, pancreas, esophagus, uterus, and breast as well on this list of stress-related disorders.

Another reaction that occurs in our bodies as a direct result of stress is inflammation. On a chronic basis, your body becomes more and more inflamed as a result of the stress that you have been experiencing. This inflammation causes other diseases and disorders. Any disease that you have been diagnosed with ending in -itis is an inflammatory condition of a specific region of the body. These specific conditions will all be helped or corrected by dealing with the underlying chronic stress response that is stimulating or aggravating that condition. Examples of these -itis conditions include arthritis, colitis, and dermatitis. These are all inflammatory conditions. Certainly, some of these can be bacterially related, such as cellulitis; however, if the overall inflammatory load in your body and immune function of your body is not adversely altered, your body can and will deal with even these immunological stressors, such as a bacterial infections, much more readily.

We think of stress as some kind of a psychic, ephemeral process that you can't really wrap your head around. It's important that we understand the process and progression of stress because there are external environmental stressors. These may involve situations, relationships, people, and experiences that occur to which we react. The react part of this equation is the critical piece of the stress puzzle to understand. How then do we as humans mentally, physically, and physiologically react to an external stressor in our environment? We may often internalize that stress, and what occurs as a result to our bodies and our physiology can be devastating to our overall health and wellness.

We have an area in the brain called the hippocampus, which is where we interpret emotions and emotional situations. That interpretation becomes physiological when a small gland right in the center of the brain, called the hypothalamus, secretes a hormone. That hormone stimulates another slightly larger gland that is located next to it, called the pituitary gland, to secrete other hormones. There can also be a direct neurological stimulation of the adrenal glands from the pituitary gland. You have two adrenal glands located right on top of your kidneys. So, what your body just did was move a signal from an area deep in your brain to a gland located in your brain, then on to another gland located near your lower back. Next, these adrenal glands, which are located a meter from the brain, produce adrenal hormones, including cortisol and adrenaline. These hormones then circulate into the body and cause the physiological changes, including increased heart rate, increased blood pressure, decreased sex drive, and decreased immune function.

Now let's take a look at these effects individually. Let's start out by looking at your heart rate. We must always ask ourselves why this type of change, in this case an elevation of your heart rate, is a good thing. Remember that your body is anticipating an acute or short-term stressor. Your body/mind knows that you are going to be running or fighting. It, therefore, wants to create the maximum blood flow so that all of the muscles are oxygenated and ready.

Why would your blood pressure go up? Why is the blood that's circulating in your body diverted from your GI tract to your extremities? You need to run or fight. You do not need to digest food, and therefore, the available blood supply is pulled from unnecessary areas and shunted to the main areas of need, in this case the extremities. Think about what happens to your digestion when you are under stress. It's suppressed, which means you cannot digest your food correctly. People get diarrhea, they vomit; all kinds of things happen to people when they're under stress to expel their gastric contents. Because you may not survive, you are not going to need to digest food at that moment. You can eat again later if you survive. The important thing that your body is trying to facilitate is your survival.

These changes that your body makes are perfect for you to deal with an acute or short-term stressor. When the stress remains for an extended period of time, you can see how the changes that the body makes in our physiology become counterproductive and disease producing.

Now, what do most of us do as a result of these changes that occur to our physiology due to these chronic stress syndromes? We run to the doctor because we have diarrhea, so they give you Imodium, for example. The medication stops the diarrhea, but it doesn't change a thing physiologically.

It should be clear to you by now why I do not separate the brain from the body. They are one integral functioning system. The mistake we made in years gone by was that we tried to segment the body. You cannot separate the body into component parts for analysis and expect to have a full grasp of how that body functions as a whole. As an example of this, you cannot separate the brain and the nervous system from the heart because they're all one when they're functioning correctly. The brain responds to physiological stressors too, by causing the release of specific hormones that alter the way that the body's systems function. These systems include, among others, your immune system. Let's say that you have a sub-clinical viral infection in your system, meaning an infection that is not affecting your blood work. Your immune system may have been fighting these viral invaders for days, weeks, or even years, but then suddenly your immune system is suppressed by chronic stress and you suddenly and unexpectedly get sick. This immune response to stress is facilitated through both hormonal changes and neurologic stimulation. This specific field of study is called psychoneuroimmunology, and it is a very fast growing field of research.

A great deal of this research is being performed at the National Institutes of Health. Thanks in great part to this ongoing research, we are now gaining an understanding of how the psyche (the brain's thoughts) affects the neuro (the nervous system) and thereby the immune system. One study indicates that chronically unhappy nurses have more episodes of cold sores than others who have already been infected with the same viral type, namely herpes simplex 1 virus. Their immune systems are suppressed by their unhappiness.

Matt Ridley published another interesting study in his book *Genome*. This is truly a fascinating book on the subject of genetics. He references a long-term study of 17,000 civil servants. The study found that the status of a person's job was a better predictor of the likelihood of a heart attack than was obesity, smoking, or high blood pressure. The findings indicate that individuals in what were ranked as low-grade jobs, for example, a janitor or custodian, were nearly four times more likely to have a heart attack than was a permanent secretary at the top of the socioeconomic structure of a business. Even if this secretary was overweight, had high blood pressure, and smoked, she was less likely to suffer from a heart attack at a given age than the janitor or custodian in the same building. The findings of this study indicate that where you are in the pecking order of a company or a business has more impact on your potential for cardiovascular disease than does your lifestyle or some of the other variables that we normally equate with heart disease and early death. Another critical and interesting finding that came out of this same study was that being in a position where you have fewer emotional stressors allows you to live a longer, healthier life.

This also correlates with death rates after retirement. Many people who retire from their jobs will end up contracting a variety of diseases and disorders and ultimately have an earlier loss of life than they would have, statistically, had they continued to work. Some of this change, if not most of it, may be due to the fact that these people no longer receive the good stress, or eustress, from their daily life experiences. They don't have to worry about getting something done in a particular day, because tomorrow will always be Saturday for them. But while we all dream of that opportunity to have every day be Saturday, there's something to be said for being busy and having control over events occurring around us.

The same thing applies to students who have experienced stressful periods. A student will be under a long period of stress, say for final exams. They may get through them fine. As soon as the exams are over, however, they become ill. They have pushed and pushed and pushed using the adrenal hormones to keep their bodies going during the final exam period. Then after that period is over, all of the things that occur due to the physiological response to stress take hold. Their immune system, which has been suppressed, suddenly becomes overwhelmed, and they become sick.

We can see this same scenario playing out by statistics on the health of folks who are unemployed. There are studies that indicate that an individual who is unemployed is more likely to become depressed and will become ill more frequently.

The effect of stress on your body/mind cannot and must not be underestimated in your quest for health and wellness.

The questions then becomes these: Is our behavior at the mercy of our biology, or is our biology at the mercy of our behavior? Does how we respond affect us physically and physiologically relative to our stressors? In other words, is what we experience in the environment the trigger for the negative physiological changes that occur to our bodies and minds when those stressors exist for an extended period of time?

Or is the opposite, in fact, the case? In other words, do the body/mind changes from the stressors in our environment affect our behavior and thereby affect our physiological as well as our physical state?

THINK RIGHT: THE SOLUTION

> *"The body is like a piano, and happiness is like music. It is needful to have the instrument in good order."*
>
> —HENRY WARD BEECHER

I'd like to review a theory that I have on the reactionary response that we often exhibit in response to stress and the resultant stress response physiology that occurs in our body/mind. The stress response physiology occurs without any conscious thought on the part of the individual who is exposed to the stressor. Remember that we all make a conscious decision to either react or respond to a given stressor. When we react, the outcome is often damaging to us physically, physiologically, and environmentally. When we respond to a stressor, the outcome is usually more positive, not only to our body/mind but also to the psyche and physiology of those around us. Often an individual will experience an issue. That issue may be simply that the individual feels that they have done something wrong.

The Emotional Ring of Fire

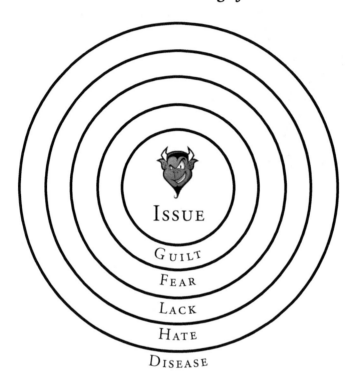

ISSUE

GUILT

FEAR

LACK

HATE

DISEASE

This wrong could have been done to themselves, the environment, or someone in their sphere of influence. Innately, we have been designed so that we have a pretty good handle on what is right and wrong. If we do something we feel is wrong or if we've wronged someone in some way, it's very difficult for us to maintain an even physiology with that wrongful event stored in our memory banks. Whether it affects us immediately or after an extended period of time, it's still there, logged away.

Over time, or sometimes immediately, that issue will create another tier of internal stress for us: the stress of guilt. This is the second layer of the cascade of reactionary response to the issue in progressive spiraling layers of the internalized stress response.

Ultimately, that guilt will create fear. Perhaps it's fear of being found out or fear that you are going to be punished. These, again, are normal, innate emotions, but they are often exaggerated. The fear we experience begins to affect our bodies negatively. As we progress through this cascade of events, you may skip levels and move more rapidly into this spiraling physiological quagmire of reactionary emotional and physical stress responses.

Next, that fear that you have of being discovered or punished will create a scenario in your mind and in your environment of lack. The lack is a mindset that occurs because you start to feel that you're not deserving of something. You have a nagging sense that you have to give something back or give something up to make up for the original issue. Much of this happens subconsciously, but you see how your original issue creates internal dialogue and internal stress, and this begins compounding the internal physiological stressors and changes in your body and mind that will negatively affect your health and wellness.

At the next layer, you will begin to experience a turnaround. This is almost a defensive method of dealing with this fear and lack that you have created. What occurs next is the development of hate. That hatred is often directed at something that has nothing to do with that initial issue. Sometimes the person or situation that you are transferring your reaction to may not be directly related to the issue. This transference of anger and hate often occurs without any conscious thought or understanding. You may begin attacking a spouse or loved one for no apparent reason.

Let's talk about how this hate manifests itself. We begin to despise a person, place, or thing that we relate to this cascade of events steaming from the initial issue. You may have resentment toward yourself. Perhaps on a subconscious or even on a conscious plane, you can't believe that you would be able to do what you've done or say what you said. Mind you, these don't have to be major issues. They just need to be big enough to trigger the cascade. You continue to have this internal dialogue about what you said to Aunt Betty last week or what you said to your boss, and now you're thinking: "Maybe I shouldn't have said that or in that way." You turn that external situation into resentment against a specific person that you relate to the incident, or perhaps a person, place, or thing that has no direct link to the original event. This is where you will start to see the physiological changes from stress compounded.

These physiological changes will cause *dis*-ease, or a lack of smooth flow in the body's systems. You might get sick more often or miss more days of work due to physical complaints, fatigue, or mental fog. That could be another way that you are compensating for what you've done. At this point, you don't necessarily see the stressor as you did before. You may even forget about it or no longer dwell on the initial issue. You are now beginning the next tier in the downward spiral of the stress cascade, which is out of your control. This next layer is now what the medical community will label a disease. This layer of disease may manifest as high blood pressure or heart disease, diabetes, cancer, strokes, and all manner of other illnesses that can be traced to the cascade of events.

The key in avoiding the ultimate end point—disease—is for you to understand where it came from and the process and progression that occurred to get you to the place where you are now. The critical skill that you must develop to cope with this situation is to recognize that you, and only you, may have created the reaction that you have had, and most, if not all, of this process occurs in your own mind. You must accept personal responsibility. Only then can you begin the steps necessary to deal with the situation and ultimately the initial issue. Dealing with it constructively and decisively is going to require meaningful change on your part. Change is often a way into a stressful situation, and change will be the way out of that same stress-producing situation. Change in and of itself can create a state of fear and further stress, but that is often the only way to dig yourself out of the spiraling cascade of events.

So what do you have to do to deal with your current situation? First, forgive—and this might start with forgiving yourself. You may have to forgive someone else. You've got to act on this one as soon as possible. Life is short, and you might not get another opportunity. You also have to realize what you are doing to yourself and others by not forgiving, by not changing, by not letting go and not taking charge. Letting go and taking charge sound like opposites, but you must take charge to let go, and you must let go to take charge.

Take responsibility and create the change that is necessary to become healthier and happier. You may need to remove the hate or that initial phase of lack. Perhaps you have developed fears or phobias. You may have guilt for something for which you can't even remember the cause. You must deal with the issue by forgiving and letting go. Just write the letter, make the phone call, and be done with it.

Ultimately, it's not going to make any difference when you're on your deathbed. I've been with enough people who have been on their death beds to state that they are not lying there thinking, "I could have made that extra $100,000," or "I could have had that job," or "I should have bought that car." It all means nothing at that point. If you let go, forgive, get over it, take charge, and create the necessary change, then you can and will move on with your life. You will be happier, much healthier, and I can guarantee you that you will add years to your life and life to your years. If you do not act on it, you are going to stay stuck right where you are. Seek help with the process if necessary. The important thing is that you move forward, so get moving.

METABOLIC SYNDROME

"It is sad to admit that our current genetically incongruent diet in the United States is referred to as the S.A.D., or the Standard American Diet."

—DR. DOUGLAS G. PFEIFFER.

I talked earlier about the explosion in diagnoses of metabolic syndrome and how it's related to our tendency as a society to not eat right, move right, think right, or sleep right. So, what is done medically for it in our current disease and sickness care system? We have developed numerous drugs to treat the symptoms of metabolic syndrome. For example, hypertension is treated medically with antihypertensive drugs, which are very commonly prescribed to anyone who has a blood pressure in excess of 140/90.

One of the most prevalent components of metabolic syndrome is elevated blood sugar levels, or type II diabetes. Years ago, the allowable fasting blood sugar levels where 140ng/dL. Today, however, the maximum allowable level of fasting blood sugar is 100ng/dL. The rate of diabetes is on the rise. Even children have elevated blood sugar levels and are being diagnosed with diabetes at an alarmingly high rate. Diabetes is the most preventable disorder. We just need to make the appropriate changes. By making these changes, we can avoid another class of oral and injectable drugs.

We've discussed another commonly prescribed class of drugs called statins, which are used to treat hypercholesterolemia, or high cholesterol levels in the blood. The pharmaceutical industry has not yet developed a feasible drug to treat obesity, but they are working on it. They have, however, developed numerous surgical procedures to treat obesity such as a lap band surgery, which is used to constrain the dimensions of the stomach so that it can't expand as much and, consequently, you can't eat as much. As a result of this procedure, you will lose weight. This surgical procedure is a very extreme one and should only be used in cases of morbid obesity where nothing else has worked.

We at the Center for Nutrition and Wellness hold a biannual cleanse event. I call it my Full System Detox Cleanse Program. I have had numerous individuals enrolled in this program. In one class of 23 participants, the calculated weight loss for the group, after only five days since initiating their lifestyle changes, was 112 pounds. Essentially, the group lost one of their members in terms of weight. Granted, it would have had to be a slender member, but 112 pounds in five days is an indication that what I teach my patients does work. By altering your lifestyle and not going down the road of drugs or surgery to deal with the complications and symptoms of metabolic syndrome, you can reverse the condition and divert your life path and your overall paradigm from the disease and sickness path to the health and wellness path in a relatively short period of time.

There is another reason I believe that avoiding these medical treatments for metabolic syndrome is so important: the side effects that each one of these drugs has on both your physiology and your overall health and wellness. Yes, it's true that if you take a statin drug for high cholesterol it will, in most instances, drive your cholesterol reading down on your next blood test. However, that does not mean that you are healthy or well. It means that you have a lower cholesterol level on a blood test.

You can artificially drive your blood pressure down, but that does nothing to decrease the inflammatory process that's occurring inside your blood vessels because both your high blood pressure and your high cholesterol are a result of the poor lifestyle choices you have made. By not eating, moving, sleeping, or thinking right, you can and do create an environment in your body that will perpetuate the disease and sickness that pervades our culture. Stress causes alterations in your heart rate, blood pressure, and inflammatory load. These changes then trigger significant physiological alterations that will lead to the onset of diseases and disorders such as diabetes, heart disease, stroke, and cancer. The choices that you make are significant ones; they will alter the course of your life and longevity.

Obviously, not only the quantity of your life, but also the quality of life will suffer once you start to manifest the secondary effects of metabolic syndrome. You will no longer be able to participate in many events and activities. You will find that your body will stop performing as well.

We'll now look at what specific things you need to do to change the course of your life. There are identifiable components of our health and wellness paradigm that you will need to begin adding, as well as choices that you will need to alter or remove from your current lifestyle to begin diverting your life's path. One good example of a change that you should make immediately relates to one of the components of metabolic syndrome: hypertension, or high blood pressure. By changing your lifestyle, beginning to incorporate some gradual and progressive exercise, and altering your stress level, you can make positive changes in your blood pressure. You can also add some nutritional supplementation to your daily regimen to support your adrenal glands. These tiny, walnut-sized glands sit on top of your kidneys and produce hormones to deal with stress, among their other functions. These tiny glands become overworked and fatigued as a result of chronic stress, because they have been overproducing stress hormones, in most instances, for years.

You can reverse this process. I've done it and I have seen many of my patients do this. Some of my patients who have been on blood pressure, diabetes, or cholesterol drugs have come into our center for help. We have been able reverse this process and assist thousands in changing their lifestyles and creating healthier lives. After they undergo an evaluation, I can determine what lifestyle changes and nutritional support are necessary to assist them in compensating for their many deficiencies and in reducing their toxicities. I use many procedures to accomplish these goals, including targeted functional nutrition. In this way, we can enhance the altered function of certain glands, organs, and tissues in the body.

Our patients who have made lifestyle changes, such as increasing their exercise level or increasing the quality of the food that they consume and the quantity and quality of their sleep, have reversed the progressive deterioration of the body, which is associated with metabolic syndrome. These patients who may be currently medicated for hypertension, as an example, often will begin to experience difficulties such as lightheadedness, perhaps some fatigue upon standing, and dizziness when they get out of bed. These are indications that the individual must go back and see their prescribing doctor to have their blood pressure medication adjusted. As the body heals and moves into a state of wellness, these patients don't require as much of the drug. Often, they no longer need the drug at all. It can be challenging; if you are not coached through the process and don't understand what is going on as you heal, you might actually think that there is something wrong when these changes occur. In fact, these changes are very positive ones, and they are an indication that something good is happening to and in your body.

I make similar changes to positively affect patients' high cholesterol levels as well. Remember, the two primary things that will increase your cholesterol level are saturated fats and sugars. Most of the time, we forget about the second component in this equation. We always focus on the saturated fat component. People try to avoid consuming fat and, in the process, often because they're compensating for a loss of flavor in their food, they end up adding sugar to their diet. There are really three things that you taste and which food processors juggle to create a food that you find appealing: fat, sugar, and salt. If a food product processor decreases the amount of fat in a specific food product, they generally will increase the quantity of sugar. The food product processors are very good at this juggling act.

Recognizing these facts, I have to be watchful when a patient is going through the process of improving their eating habits to make sure they are not compensating when we reduce sugar intake. What I mean by the term compensating is that I have to make sure that the individual is not increasing saturated fat intake to compensate for a lack of flavor due to the reduction in sugar in the food they are consuming. By monitoring those two contributing factors to hypercholesterolemia, namely the consumption of sugar and saturated fat, in concert with increasing exercise levels, I have been able to cause a significant reduction in total cholesterol levels. This means there is not only a reduction in LDL cholesterol, but also a concurrent increase in HDL cholesterol.

If a patient has a significantly elevated blood cholesterol level, I will incorporate some specific nutritional supplementation. These supplements may include things such as coenzyme Q10 or red yeast rice as well as omega-3 fatty acids in the form of fish oil. I include these supplements when the cholesterol level is exceptionally high because frequently a patient will be deficient in these essential nutrients, particularly the CoQ10, and the omega-3s. Most everyone is deficient in omega-3 fatty acids and toxic in omega-6 fatty acids because of the quantity of grain-based food products that they consume on a daily basis. While omega-6 fats are a necessary nutrient, they are also inflammatory. Because our diets have been toxic in grains, we have become toxic in omega-6 fats, and therefore, the inflammatory load in the body of the average American has also increased. By supplementing omega-3 fatty acids and reducing the quantity of grains in a patient's diet, I will not only create a better ratio of omega-3 to omega-6 fatty acids, but I will see a concurrent reduction in the patient's total cholesterol levels as well.

Coenzyme Q10 is something I usually recommend to patients who are on or just coming off of statin drugs. We use it to reduce cholesterol levels, but it is also an essential nutrient that is typically required by anyone taking a statin drug. I will routinely make sure that these patients are supplementing with coenzyme Q10. Coenzyme Q10 is a substance that's found in every cell in our body. It's used in the mitochondria, or the energy-generating portion of the cell, to generate energy in the form of adenosine triphosphate (ATP), which is used by every tissue in our bodies as an energy source. We must have sufficient production of ATP to maintain mental and physical stability.

Statin drugs deplete coenzyme Q10 in the body systemically. When this occurs, you experience a subsequent reduction in energy production. If this reduction in energy production becomes significant enough, it will cause alterations in muscle function to the point where muscle deterioration can result. If this process continues long enough, it can cause irreparable damage to the muscle tissue. While that outcome is infrequent, it is a secondary effect that can occur when statin drugs are used for a prolonged period of time.

Another key component that I strongly recommend you add to your daily routine that will affect virtually every component of metabolic syndrome is exercise. Eating correctly is essential; a vegetable-based diet with some nuts, fruits, and meats, specifically fish and poultry, will enhance your outcome in controlling metabolic syndrome. Getting a sufficient quantity and quality of sleep will also help in correcting this condition. I always encourage my patients to do this without resorting to commonly prescribed drugs.

This metabolic syndrome conundrum is a downward spiraling process that can be altered through appropriate lifestyle changes.

Unfortunately, this is all too often not done. The scenario that I see usually starts with one or two drugs and then progresses on to more and more drugs. The condition is typically treated in a way that does virtually nothing to correct the root causes of the condition. Instead, the medical profession treats the symptoms by using drugs that will force the body to move in a direction that does not necessarily create health and wellness, but creates better numbers on your blood work. Just because you have lowered your cholesterol levels does not mean that you will live a longer or healthier life. Just because your blood pressure is driven lower by prescription drugs does not necessarily enhance your overall longevity.

This is especially true when the side effects of these drugs are factored into the equation. The secondary effects of many of the drugs that are commonly prescribed for metabolic syndrome can be significant relative to your overall health and wellness. I am certainly not telling you that you should discontinue these drugs without proper recommendations and supervision, along with the consent of your prescribing doctor. If there can be a properly supervised reduction in these drugs following significant, progressive alterations in your daily lifestyle choices, you will feel better mentally as well as physically. Along with this, you will also experience that your overall health and wellness and longevity can and will be enhanced too.

I encourage you to begin the process of reversing metabolic syndrome, using the simple, if sometimes challenging, lifestyle changes I've outlined. These simple changes will, in a relatively short period of time, change not only your blood pressure readings, your cholesterol level, and your weight, but they will also change your life path from the disease and sickness paradigm to the health and wellness paradigm. This is a logical and hopefully understandable way to treat these conditions and move you forward in your quest to live a longer, healthier life.

WOMEN'S HEALTH

> *"Lack of activity destroys the good condition of every human being, while movement and methodical physical exercise save it and preserve it."*

—PLATO

There are very few of us who have not been affected by cancer, whether it is personally or through a family member or a friend. Breast cancer is one of the most common forms of cancer today and has touched the lives of virtually everyone. While there are numerous causes of breast cancer, from genetic predisposition to environmental factors, there are also specific lifestyle decisions that you can make that will reduce your potential for acquiring this devastating form of cancer. Simply having the BRCA1 and BRCA2 genes (the breast cancer genes) does not necessarily mean that you will get breast cancer. By incorporating appropriate lifestyle choices and activities in your eat right, think right, move right, and sleep right pillars of health, you can down-regulate the breast cancer gene. This means that you can significantly reduce the likelihood that this gene will express itself. Doing the correct things gives you a significant degree of control over whether these genes will turn on.

One of those things is to exercise. Exercise creates alterations in hormone levels. By exercising appropriately, you can enhance immune function to assist you in fighting off any form of cancer you encounter. Every one of us is exposed to different invaders in our daily routines, such as bacteria and viruses that are trying to proliferate in our bodies. They can then set up shop, so to speak, and begin to propagate in an attempt to overwhelm our bodies' natural defenses. If this happens, the alterations that occur on a cellular level can be enough to move us toward a state of immune overload and set us up for cancerous growth and proliferation due to this immune overload. However, we are designed with built-in defense mechanisms.

These mechanisms involve the ability of our own immune system to kill off those invaders, whether they are viral or bacterial, fungal or parasitic. In essence, we are successfully fighting cancer every day by having a fully functioning immune system. You enhance your immune system's ability to do its job correctly by exercising, eating appropriately, getting enough healthful rest, and reducing emotional and psychophysiologic stress. There are specific foods that are beneficial to all of us and that should be consumed on a routine basis, but definitely by women, because these foods help to support, for example, breast health.

The first on that list are cruciferous vegetables, which are sulfur-containing foods. Examples of these would be cabbage, broccoli, cauliflower, kale, and kohlrabi. Brussels sprouts are another example, as are turnips, collards, and rutabaga. Cruciferous vegetables contain a substance called indole-3-carbinol (I3C). I3C is converted in your body into another substance called diindolylmethane (DIM). The importance of these two chemical substances is that they assist in the reduction of estrogen levels in the body. The quantity of estrogen in your body can cause an up-regulation of cancer-producing genes. By reducing the quantity of estrogen in your system, you can reduce the potential for turning on those genes or causing breast cancer to occur in the first place.

There are two ways in which I3C and DIM affect your body's estrogen level. First, they affect it by improving the way in which your body metabolizes estrogen; in other words, the way it gets estrogen out of your system. Generally, this occurs in the liver and I3C enhances this process of cleaning estrogen out of your system in this manner. The second way that these two substances assist in avoiding the onset of breast cancer is by improving the function of tumor-suppressing genes.

As an added bonus, these two substances also block cancer-causing chemicals, including estrogen, from attaching to estrogen receptor sites on the breast tissue. What are estrogen receptor sites? Imagine a lock and key: estrogen-receptor sites are the lock, and the key would be the estrogen itself that fits into the lock. DIM and IC3 mimic estrogen, and therefore, they'll fit into the lock equally well as the estrogen key. In doing so, they block the estrogen from attaching to estrogen-receptor sites in the breast and reduce the potential that the breast tissue will turn cancerous.

By eating these sulfur-containing, cruciferous vegetables, you will increase your IC3 and, ultimately, DIM quantities which reduce the potential for the conversion of cells that are normal and healthy in your breast into cancerous cells. You will also decrease your overall estrogen load. Oftentimes, as women progress through the middle portion of their life and enter into menopause, they become estrogen dominant. They may develop extremely high concentrations of estrogen circulating in their bodies. This high concentration enhances the mutation of normal, healthy cells into cancerous cells. You will decrease your estrogen-dominant state by increasing the consumption of these types of vegetables.

Sleep is extremely important in this regard as well. Reduction of stress is crucial in reducing your potential conversion from normal, healthy tissue to cancerous tissue. Everyone understands that routine screening by physical examination is one of the best ways to screen for cancer. Arguably, mammograms do detect breast cancer; however, I want you to understand that this method does nothing to prevent breast cancer, because by the time breast cancer is identified on a mammogram it is already there.

The only confirmed cause of breast cancer is radiation from a radiographic (radiation) technique. According to one study, every mammogram you have increases your statistical risk of being diagnosed with breast cancer by 1 percent. If you were to have one mammogram per year starting at age 40, you would have increased your likelihood of getting breast cancer by 10 percent by age 50. This technique (a mammogram) along with most, if not all, other medical diagnostic techniques are early detection techniques, not preventative techniques. Another problem with mammograms is their high percentages of false positive results as well as false negatives. The results of a study published in 2012, "General Health Checks in Adults for Reducing Morbidity and Mortality from Disease,"[4] indicate that even routine screenings

---

4   Lasse T. Krogsboll, et. al., "General Health Checks in Adults for Reducing Morbidity and Mortality from Disease: Cochrane Systematic Review and Meta-analysis," *BMJ*, (2012), E7191, doi: 10.1002/14651858.CD009009.pub2.

such as mammograms do virtually nothing to reduce mortality rates.

My focus is to encourage you to do things to truly prevent the onset of breast cancer, along with many other disorders. Continue your self-examinations and get your regular checkups and learn about other techniques for monitoring breast health, including thermography and MRI scans, which involve no radiation of the breast tissue. These techniques will be incorporated into the mainstream in the not too distant future, because they pose little to no known health risk for patients and can be much more sensitive to detecting breast cancer. Because of this, they can detect changes in the breast tissue much earlier. For you to be proactive in truly preventing breast cancer, as you must be with all other disorders, you need to begin incorporating the necessary lifestyle changes.

Thyroid disorders affect many women and men. The thyroid gland is an important gland in our bodies because it regulates so many functions. It controls our metabolism. It will cause weight gain or weight loss, depending on whether it is functioning in a hypo or hyper state. It will cause alterations in heart rate and in body temperature. It's something that is often initially overlooked when patients have complaints related to these types of symptoms.

The function of the thyroid gland is affected to a significant degree by iodine levels in our bodies. Iodine is a mineral that is required in small quantities for the thyroid gland to function correctly. Iodine is important to the function of many other glands, organs, and tissues as well. There are iodine receptors on various sex glands and breast tissue. The primary gland and tissue that we think of when iodine is discussed is the thyroid gland, and rightfully so, because iodine is required for the production of thyroid hormones. If insufficient iodine is available, that hormone production will be significantly reduced.

In the first decade of the 20th century, particularly in the Midwestern states, the percentage of individuals who developed goiters began increasing significantly. A goiter is an excessive growth of the thyroid gland to the point where it is often visibly noticeable at the base of the neck. If you have ever seen someone with a goiter, it's impossible to miss. Some goiters can become so large that they extend down below the breastbone internally.

The federal government recognized that the reason people were developing these goiters was because they were deficient in iodine. They decided that it would be necessary to supplement some food that the population consumed on a routine basis with iodine. The decision was made to supplement salt. That is why in the 1920s, we began iodizing salt. By doing so, the federal government temporarily stemmed the epidemic of thyroid goiter formation.

You can see the quandary that many people who have high blood pressure face because they've been instructed to reduce salt intake. By reducing salt intake, you concurrently reduce your iodine intake. We have now reached a point where many people are iodine deficient and never know it. We now have a culture in which the fourth leading prescribed drug is levothyroxine, the generic form of Synthroid. The name brand Synthroid was coined from synthetic thyroid hormone. Statistically, an underactive thyroid gland or hypothyroidism is much more common than an overactive thyroid gland. The medical community will use this synthetic thyroxin (thyroid hormone) or Synthroid to treat the condition. In the scenario of hypothyroidism, a thyroid gland is not producing enough thyroid hormone. In the current medical system, the answer to hypothyroidism is to supplement with a synthetic thyroid hormone to compensate.

Now, here are the concerns that we face with this method of treatment. We are doing absolutely nothing to treat the cause of the condition. Synthroid does not cause a specific positive alteration in the function of the thyroid gland. It essentially compensates for the lack of function of the thyroid gland, at least in the case of a patient who has a low-functioning thyroid or a hypothyroid condition. What is actually occurring is that the thyroid gland stops functioning correctly. There can be numerous causes for this lack of function. However, in the medical system we choose to merely orally administer the hormone that is not being produced by that gland. No specific consideration is given to the question of why the thyroid gland is not producing enough of the hormone. The philosophy is to simply compensate for the lack of production. This may seem like a logical thing to do, but let's look a little further into the result of this treatment.

How does the body react to the administration of synthetic thyroid hormone? The body will do a chemical analysis, which it does every nanosecond, to determine what hormones need to be produced, what substances there are too much of or not enough of. Now all of a sudden, your body is getting thyroid hormone that's being ingested. It doesn't necessarily recognize whether the thyroid is producing it or not. What does that do to your thyroid gland? It reduces the thyroid gland's natural production of thyroid hormones.

If your thyroid gland was not producing enough thyroid hormone and you supplement your body artificially with a form of the thyroid hormone that is already deficient, your body will recognize that there is now enough thyroid hormone circulating in the blood stream. As a result of this, the brain will actually cause a reduction in natural production of thyroid hormone. Thus, in this all-too-common scenario, the cause of this problem is ignored. Rather, it is circumvented by supplying the body with synthetic hormones, making the problem of your body's natural production of thyroid hormones worse.

Many of you may be on Synthroid or levothyroxine, but I want you to recognize that when you supplement with a hormone like Synthroid, there can be no alteration. Your dose is your dose. You take the same amount every day. There is no increase or decrease in production based on the body's needs. Consequently, your body doesn't function as optimally as it could if thyroid hormone production were enhanced as opposed to being compensated for. Our goal should be to enhance the production when possible.

What do we do about the lack of production in the first place? Well, let's go back to what happened in the 1920s. I said that people didn't receive enough iodine in their diets so their thyroid gland grew larger. Why would the body cause the thyroid gland to grow larger? Because the thyroid gland is not producing enough thyroid hormone at its current size, the body enlarges the gland so that it can produce more thyroid hormone. The hypertrophy, or overgrowth, of that thyroid gland is a natural way for your body to enhance the production of the thyroid hormone. What is the root of that problem? Your body is not able to produce enough thyroid hormone because it doesn't have enough raw materials. In this case, the missing raw material may be iodine. At the Center, we often use oral iodine administration to naturally enhance thyroid function.

There are competitive binders for iodine in this process as well, which further complicates the situation. You will remember that when we reviewed estrogen binding to breast cells, I described it as being like a lock and key. There are similar iodine-binding sites on the thyroid gland. They also function like the lock, and the iodine is the right key to fit into that lock. There are other elements, however, that closely resemble iodine.

If you remember the periodic chart of elements, you may know that there were other elements that are in the same elemental group as iodine. They are called halides. The halides include such things as bromine, fluorine, and chlorine. They have the ability to enter into our body, and they mimic iodine. They will bind to iodine-receptor sites. The chlorine that you use to wash your whites in your laundry is one of those halides. It is absorbed through the skin, just like the chlorine that you use to clean your sink, which is also absorbed through the skin. So is the fluoride toothpaste that you use to brush your teeth, which is absorbed through the mucous membranes of your mouth and enters into your body in this way. Today, the mass-produced bread we eat has bromine. It binds to the iodine-binding sites on your thyroid gland when insufficient iodine is taken in. However, they cannot be used to produce thyroid hormones like iodine.

When we supplement a patient with iodine at the Center for Nutrition and Wellness, I find that the patient may have a "kick off." Here's what happens: The binding sites on the thyroid gland have the ability to recognize when iodine is available and in close proximity. The binding locations on the thyroid gland can actually recognize that the iodine is what should be preferentially bound to these sites. The fluorine, chlorine, and bromine will then be "kicked off" of the thyroid gland, and the iodine will then bind to those sites. When that occurs, a patient may develop excessive amounts of these other halide substances. The body wants to rid itself of these other halides as efficiently and rapidly as it can. This may mean that the only route left is for these halides to be pushed out through the skin. It's not uncommon when we start supplementing a patient with iodine that they have a rash or an irritation on the skin.

Iodine deficiency is an often overlooked cause of altered thyroid function. It sounds like a simple solution to a large problem that is rampant throughout our culture. The solution is usually a change in lifestyle to compensate for a deficiency or a toxicity. These are generally not difficult changes to make, particularly when the changes are viewed as the pathway to health and wellness. But each of these changes has its own challenges, especially because most of us live around other well-intentioned people who may not be as well informed.

Recently, I had an opportunity to speak with one of my patients who is going through our full system detox cleanse. She told me that when people looked at how she was eating or the supplementation that she was taking, they were uncomfortable with these changes because they are not the status quo. These positive lifestyle changes definitely will lead her down a different path. That different path may be very challenging to those well-intentioned individuals in your sphere of influence because these changes are foreign to them and even a little scary. Change is always challenging, and when friends and family indirectly experience those changes, it creates unrest in them because you are becoming a different person both physically, mentally, and oftentimes spiritually.

By living a genetically congruent lifestyle and having your friends and family witness the changes that you are making and their effects, they will want to become a part of those changes and this new paradigm that you are creating. As you start changing your lifestyle, you will find that the people in your sphere of influence may comment about what you are doing. People may inadvertently make you feel awkward. You have to be strong enough in your belief and your desire to make these changes so you can overlook those comments. Remember that the individuals who are saying these things are usually well intentioned. Unfortunately, they are ignorant regarding the information that you are learning and incorporating into your psyche and your lifestyle.

Be patient and nurture them; you may be surprised by how they gradually begin to join you on your journey. You can and will be an example for others. Sometimes, that means that you have to use the practices discussed in the stress section of this book. For example, you may need to just laugh or make a joke out of what they are saying. You cannot take it personally because if you do it's going to derail your progress and your movement toward your genetically congruent lifestyle.

CHAPTER 5

MOVE RIGHT: THE CHALLENGE

"Those who think they have not time for bodily exercise will sooner or later have to find time for illness."

—EDWARD SMITH-STANLEY

G ood health requires movement, but as a society, we simply don't move enough. In our culture, our habit of movement has degraded from the way we were genetically designed to move. Our Paleolithic ancestors were physically very active, migrating on average about ten miles a day. During that day, they would perform a variety of motions, including jumping, bending, twisting, and climbing to acquire foodstuffs for themselves and the members of their tribes.

Today, we are required to do very little moving, and many of us avoid it at all costs. Just look at people in a mall or supermarket parking lot who will almost battle over snagging the parking space that's closest to the doors. Our lifestyles are largely sedentary, both in our work and in our leisure activities. At work, we sit in front of the computer screen or perform duties that are very repetitive and routine. Then we come home, eat dinner, and sit down to watch television for hours on end.

We have come to a point where we have recognized this lack of exercise and we are trying to compensate for it. Unfortunately, in many instances we are overcompensating. This unnaturally sedentary lifestyle has created a variety of disorders. It is unfortunate that we have begun to define deficiency syndromes as actual diseases. Conditions including increased cholesterol, obesity, heart disease, increased blood pressure, and even stroke, diabetes, and cancer can all be related to a lack of movement and motion. This lack of movement is one integral part of the health and wellness paradigm.

The lack of motion can occur on a gross or systemic level where we are just not moving our bodies enough, or on a minute, or segmental, level. I deal with both on a daily basis where this lack of motion relates to spinal disorders. The key to solving this problem is to first recognize our lack of motion and mobility. The problem is that oftentimes we don't recognize it until it is almost too late. Consequently, we get into a mode where the lack of motion and mobility creates secondary problems that compound that lack of motion and mobility. The most obvious effect of this is obesity. Once you're obese, you don't want to move, because it is such an effort. That mass that you have developed becomes a great deterrent to motion. This cycle becomes self-perpetuating as time goes on.

Unfortunately, many folks start experiencing the secondary issues of this lack of motion and mobility, like having high blood pressure. By using drugs in an attempt to correct the problem, they are artificially lowering those numbers, while doing nothing to increase their overall health and wellness.

When I discuss any type of degenerative change in a joint with a patient, I always use the analogy of a rusty hinge. As time goes on and the hinge progressively rusts and degenerates, it won't move as far, so we don't open the gate quite as far. Over time, that rust insidiously increases, just like the degenerative change in a joint progressively worsens with less and less movement. The flip side is that you can increase mobility in a joint just like oiling and moving a hinge. Much like that rusty hinge, we may not be able to bring the joint back to as good as new, but we can create better function than it currently has.

The other consequence is the neurological health that motion creates. Every joint in your body has nerve receptors embedded in it and in the surrounding tissues. The muscles, tendons, and ligaments all have nerve receptors that give input to your brain and receive output from your brain. If a joint starts to break down, there are pain receptors in the joint that will start to fire and give negative input to your brain about moving that joint. Your brain starts to tell you, "Don't move the joint because it is causing pain for you." You also have balance receptors in your joints that constantly give the brain input as to what your current position is. Unfortunately, with the lack of motion, these balance receptors stop firing. You are not moving, so the receptors don't send the normal healthy input to your brain as to your current position.

To make this clearer, try an experiment: stand up, close your eyes, put your arm out to your side at ninety degrees, and wiggle your fingers. With your eyes closed, how do you know that your arm is at ninety degrees to your body and you are wiggling your fingers? You have no visual sense of that; however, you have joint receptors in every one of the joints in your hand and arm that send input to your brain to tell your brain what position that arm is in at that moment.

This input is nourishing your brain, but if you don't move, you don't get that input. Your brain and nervous system want this positive input and need it on a routine basis in order to maintain health and wellness. The brain will interpret this neurologic input and fire information to other joints and muscles to coordinate balance, posture, and your position sense. This is part of the reason that elderly people fall. Their imbalance problems are directly related to their lack of motion and the lack of nourishment to the brain from these joint receptors. When you have good, healthy nourishment going to your brain from these joint receptors, your brain will send signals to the muscles in your legs, arms, and torso to cause contractions to compensate for that alteration in your position. If you don't have that healthy joint receptor input to the brain, there is no compensatory change in the muscles and you fall.

If you don't want to get old fast, you must move! So, what do we do to get these inputs and this neurologic feedback working correctly? Your body will make neurologic changes without your even knowing it to prepare you for a stressor. It doesn't matter whether that stressor is something you are going to run away from or fight. Your body will make those necessary changes through the autonomic nervous system. If you are suddenly startled, as when someone jumps out from behind a bush and scares you, you don't consciously think, *I am going to increase my heart rate. I am going to dilate my pupils. I am going to shut down circulation to my GI tract.* It automatically happens through the autonomic nervous system, and in nanoseconds. There are autonomic nerves that run through your spine, which is how your body communicates to and from your brain about what it needs to do in relationship to what is going on in your immediate situation and in your current environment.

In the 1950s, a medical doctor by the name of Ruth Jackson did research on the cervical syndrome, which revolves around a lack of joint motion. She termed it a subluxation, or a misalignment of the vertebrate in the spine. While this was a medical doctor, not a chiropractor, she was researching and teaching one of the basic tenants of the chiropractic profession: when a vertebra becomes misaligned and locks the joint, it is no longer mobile and no longer healthy. How does this happen? Oftentimes, it is trauma that induces it, such as a whiplash injury, a fall, or perhaps a sports injury.

There are certainly numerous non-traumatic causes of this segmental joint fixation, or locking, including stress and other toxicities. Once it occurs, however, that joint no longer moves correctly. In the neck, there is a plethora of autonomic nerves exiting from the spine, particularly the division called the sympathetic division of the autonomic nervous system. The sympathetic branch is the component of the autonomic nervous system that heightens, or ramps up, your physiology. You can equate it to the gas pedal in a car. In other words, it's the part of the nervous system that causes your heart rate to go up, pupils to dilate, and blood pressure to increase automatically.

In the case of the cervical syndrome Dr. Jackson researched and wrote about, there is no stressor causing it, other than a joint that no longer moves correctly. This aberrant joint will cause a constant irritation to the sympathetic nerves that exit the spine in the neck. Doctor Jackson, being a medical doctor, presented in her book, *The Cervical Syndrome*, a great deal of information about how to diagnose the cervical syndrome through x-rays. Most of what she used for treatment was standard medical treatments, including injections into the joints and massage. Dr. Jackson found that the symptoms of cervical sympathetic irritation included increased heart rate, increased blood pressure, atrial fibrillation, along with tingling and numbness in the arms and hands.

Now, think about this for a minute: if you had this cervical syndrome occurring, and you suddenly began experiencing tingling and numbness in your left arm and hand, increased blood pressure, and heart palpitations, what are you going to do? You are going to a hospital and you are going to have a cardiac workup. And rightfully so, but the emergency room doctors may or may not find that you have some alteration in your cardiac function, because this alteration in cardiac function may in fact be caused by altered segmental joint motion in your neck irritating a sympathetic nerve and causing all of these secondary symptoms.

Truly, this is the basis for the philosophy of the chiropractic profession. Again, Dr. Jackson demonstrated that by correcting this cervical syndrome, you could correct all of these secondary symptoms. The lack of motion will cause the ultimate breakdown and degeneration of those joints. In her book, Dr. Jackson references x-rays of patients who had trauma to their neck. She shows on x-rays how the joint has been altered in its position. Subsequent x-rays of that same joint showed that the misaligned joint began to degenerate and become arthritic.

Remember, this is your body doing what it's meant to do and what is naturally right for you. The body, in its infinite wisdom, senses this lack of motion as a problem. It considers the joint to not be functioning as designed because it is not moving correctly. Because the body is a very efficient system, it will not expend energy on anything that it doesn't have to. Consequently, the body will decrease circulation to the joints that no longer move. It will cause further immobilization of the joint by laying down scar tissue, which will ultimately cause the calcification of that joint. The end result of this process of energy conservation will be bone spur formation and further degeneration of that joint. The disc in a spinal joint will break down further because it no longer gets the circulation that it once did.

Obviously, the earlier a condition such as this can be addressed, the better. Addressing it involves segmental motion, putting motion back into that joint and getting it to function the way it was designed to and the way it must function to be healthy. The key to this variety of symptoms and signs that occur as a result of the cervical syndrome is that motion has to be restored.

Perhaps you don't need a beta blocker or Neurontin for the tingling and numbness in your arm. Maybe you need to have joint mobility restored so that function returns. This neurologic component of lack of motion occurs in virtually every joint in your body. It is more commonly seen in the spinal joints because they are laden with many more nerve fibers than many other joints in the body.

Another symptom of lack of motion that is often mistakenly attributed to other causes is vertigo, the sense that everything is spinning around you. Many patients report that they wake up with this feeling for no apparent reason. They are often prescribed medications like the brand name Antivert, which is the antihistamine meclizine, to override the symptoms. One of the most common causes for vertigo is an alteration in joint motion in the neck vertebra. This lack of motion or fixation of the joint will cause altered balance input to your brain. By altering the input to the brain, the body interprets the input abnormally. The nervous system will then overcompensate, and in doing so, it creates a sense of imbalance. While vertigo can be caused by numerous other factors such as an inner ear problem or a tumor on the acoustic nerve, those causes are rarer than an abnormality in joint motion in the neck and the subsequent irritation of the nerves in the neck. When you factor this in with obesity and cardiovascular disease that lack of motion will ultimately cause, you can see how broad the disease-producing effect can be.

Your body is an intricately designed intercommunicating ecosystem; the cells communicate with one another. Most of the communication in the body occurs through the nervous system, or the endocrine or glandular systems. The brain communicates with the rest of the body through neurologic inputs and glands that cause alterations in body functions by releasing certain hormones. An example of this would be the thyroid gland, which releases a specific hormone that may cause an increase in your weight, alter your heart rate, or change other metabolic functions. This physiologic function is under the direct control and constant supervision of your nervous system. Recent research, however, has demonstrated that cells can communicate with one another through direct physical contact. The cells have fibers that extend from the nucleus, or the center point of the cell, all the way out through the cell membrane by which they can communicate with other cells around them. This communication can be sequential and progressive from one cell to another.

There is also a great deal of research that demonstrates that this cellular communication in our bodies can be altered by tissue damage or injury. A football injury, for example, where there has been a significant trauma to the thigh muscle, can cause an alteration in the tissues on a cellular level. Not only will we see a change in the communication from one cell to another, but this structural change in the cell can affect the genetic expression of the cell as well. Because these interconnecting cellular fibers extend into the nucleus of the cell where the DNA is located, the sequential physical deformation of the cells will cause the expression of the DNA to change. You can change your DNA expression through the tweaks that you can make to your lifestyle choices every day. By positively altering what you do in your daily activities, meaning what you eat and how you think and move, as well as making sure that you are getting solid, sound regenerative rest, you can reset your body's function and restore overall health and wellness.

The sequential physical deformation of cells may in some ways explain conditions like reflex sympathetic dystrophy. In this condition, an individual has what seems to be a relatively minor, innocuous trauma, which then blossoms into a myriad of diffuse and diverse symptoms that seem totally out of proportion to the initial trauma. These alterations in tissues that occur are dramatic and can be dynamic in relation to the function of our ecosystem.

MOVE RIGHT: THE SOLUTION

"Lack of activity destroys the good condition of every human being, while movement and methodical physical exercise save it and preserve it."

—PLATO

So, how do we deal with these changes? These changes can be self-perpetuating, so the first thing that you must do is to recognize that there is a problem and initiate change. Change is challenging and none of us like it, but by recognizing the issue and going outside of your comfort zone to correct it, you have begun the process of healing. The lifestyle changes will cause dramatic and observable improvement, but correcting the damage that has been done will take time. You cannot become frustrated or give up because you are not seeing immediate improvement.

Unfortunately, we live in a world of immediacy. We are looking for the pill or potion that is going to make the correction overnight. Our bodies do not heal in that way. Ultimately, the only thing that heals your body *is* your body. I don't care what medication you are given or what surgery you have had. After a surgery, your body heals itself, and it takes time. Anyone who has had a knee replacement, for instance, knows it takes months and months, often a year or two, before becoming functional again. To expect immediate results would be unrealistic, depressing, and self-defeating.

With motion, you must start the process gradually and progressively build on it. Start with the simple things: park farther away from the front door of the mall or the supermarket. If you work in a sedentary job where you sit for eight hours a day, you must get up and move on a routine basis. If you can't get up, move in your chair. Move your legs, flex and extend your feet, bend your knees, and straighten them out. Put your arm out to the side, and move it in circles, move it back and forward. Rotate your head to one side and then to the other. This is good, healthy motion, and it creates good neurological health.

The late, great fitness guru Jack Lalanne (who was himself a chiropractor) strengthened his body using a kitchen chair. He did all of his exercises by using his body weight. You don't need to spend a lot of money or buy the equipment shown on an infomercial that claims that it is going to help you get six-pack abs and lose 50 pounds in two days. You merely need to apply simple techniques that will not change your lifestyle dramatically. Just make sure that you do them on a consistent basis.

Make sure you are practicing good posture as well. One thing that occurs to us over time is "caving in." Take a look at older people; they generally began the process of caving in during their mid-life years. Their head begins to flex or tip forward; they have an anterior or forward head carriage in relation to their shoulders. Their shoulders roll forward as well. Ultimately, this will cause compression of the chest and potential cardiovascular and pulmonary problems. Once this occurs, you cannot expand your chest, and therefore, you can no longer take in a full, health-producing breath of air. Once your shoulders are rolled forward and your head tilts forward, you begin to progressively compress your torso. If, however, you recognize this process and begin to make conscious changes in this pattern, you can ward off the negative effects of caving in.

You can begin by throwing your shoulders back and holding your head in an upright posture. You will now be able to take in a deeper breath. Sit up straight when you are sitting in your chair; use the muscles at the back of your spine to hold you up. That's what they were designed to do. Those erector muscles will become weakened over time. Concurrently, the muscles in the front of your body become contracted, which is another reason that people begin to bend over forward and assume that stooped posture as they age. When you get home from work, make a concerted effort to not sit in front of the television. Go outside and take a walk. If you can't take a walk, lie on the floor to do some pelvic tilt exercises or do some abdominal crunch exercises. Obviously, you don't want to do all of these things if you are not ready for it, and it is always a good idea to consult your health care provider before you do any rigorous exercise to ensure that you are healthy enough for this type of activity.

You can start doing some simple stretches if nothing else. What does any animal do first thing in the morning when they are awakened? Unlike most of us, they stretch. All of the joints, tendons, and muscles are taut when you first wake up because you have not moved. If you get up and start moving without first stretching and limbering yourself up, you have a significantly increased potential to injure yourself. You have to first stretch those muscle fibers and joints. When you move an unhealthy joint, you may hear a clicking or popping sound. This is because the joint is moving in an almost ratcheting fashion rather than a smooth gliding fashion because of the accumulation of joint "junk". You've built up scar tissue, perhaps, or calcium deposits. But you still want to move that joint, always within the confines of pain. You don't want to force it and create more pain, but you want to maintain and build the mobility and motion in that joint. You will find over time, as you move the joint, your range of motion will increase. This occurs because motion will create increased lubrication in the joint, much like oiling and moving a rusty hinge.

Walking is a great exercise. Many people think they have to run or jog to get sufficient exercise. Macadam, concrete, and extremely hard ground can cause compression and trauma to joints in the hips, knees, and ankles. Knee, hip, ankle, and spinal injuries are frequently related to running, even in young people. The youngest patient I've seen with this kind of injury was a 16-year-old boy who had a disk herniation and degeneration in the lower back. This young man had been involved in contact sports (which most sports are today, including soccer and basketball) since he was four years old. We push high-impact sports too hard today, and children start them much too young.

Sports are not bad, neither is running, but it is important that you create a balance. Sometimes individuals are too manic in the way they exercise. You shouldn't do all of the jumping, twisting, and moving right off the bat. You need to give yourself time to get mobile before doing aggressive kinetic exercise.

Weight training is a form of exercise that is beneficial in our move right pillar of health. But this form of exercise must also be started gradually. You certainly don't want to go all in and start pumping iron right off the bat. If you're not competing for a body building contest, your body is a sufficient weight to lift. Use your body as a weight by doing some gentle, one-quarter abdominal crunches and modified pushups. There's a big selection of expensive equipment that you can buy if you would like to, but you don't have to get all the whiz-bang things to strengthen your body. Here at the Center, we've found that yoga stretching is an ideal form of exercise for most people. It creates good mobility in the joints as well as health and mobility in the connecting muscles, ligaments, and tendons that support the joints.

The main message of this chapter is to move. Your body requires it on every level for health, including neurologically. Exercise is now one of the treatments used for patients with Alzheimer's because it provides the brain with proper neurologic input and assists in reestablishing those pathways that are being lost. Movement and motion are important, not only on a gross basis, but also on a segmental basis, such as for the individual joints in the spine. I advocate for (and practice myself) regular maintenance chiropractic adjustments. This is how you can keep fixated, or locked, joints in the spine and extremities from altering the neurologic input to and output from your brain. This practice will also assist in keeping joints mobile, thereby reducing the potential of joint decay and degeneration that we commonly refer to as arthritis.

So, the next time you go to the supermarket, get out of the mind-set that you have to fight for the nearest parking space. Park a little farther away, and take a walk when you get home rather than flopping down on the couch to watch television. Start moving at work even if it is just your feet and toes.

Balance and stability are essential components of the overall health and wellness paradigm. And it is easily lost as we age. Here is one simple-to-do exercise that I recommend to many of my patients that assists them in maintaining their balance and position sense. I am confident that this procedure will aid you in your quest for postural balance as you progress through life. Stand next to a wall, a chair, or a counter top, close enough to grab it quickly, but you should not hang onto it. Raise one foot off of the ground for 30 seconds without reaching for support if you can. Then try it with the other foot. You may find that you're more stable on one leg than the other. You will also find that if you do this exercise daily, you will be able to balance yourself better as time goes on.

Individuals who do this exercise regularly, over time, can flex their entire body forward and extend their leg out behind them while maintaining balance on one leg. I am certainly not suggesting that you try this as a beginner because even a seasoned balancer must practice extreme caution when doing this. You will find, however, that as you begin regaining your balance you may have to make the process a little more challenging. As your balance improves, there are devices that you can incorporate into your exercise routine including wobble boards and exercise balls.

Motion equals health. This is a definitive and irrefutable truth. It is imperative that you recognize this to move forward in your quest for your optimal level of health and wellness. You must incorporate this pillar into your paradigm not just to maintain your longevity, but also to improve your quality of life. Chronologically, we are living longer than ever before, but our functional life span, that period of your life in which you can actually function without being dependent on others, is not keeping up. You can avoid the need for the plethora of drugs and surgical procedures that are prescribed today to treat the various symptoms. Your functional life span is about 64 years. This is in contrast to your actual life span, which is about 78 years. That means our functional life span is coming up short by about 14 years. My goal is to see that you learn right now what you can do to live, and not just exist.

CHAPTER 6

SLEEP RIGHT

"Early to bed and early to rise, makes a man
healthy, wealthy and wise."

—BENJAMIN FRANKLIN

For many people, particularly as they hit middle age, sleep becomes a real health and wellness issue, both to its quality and quantity. Duration of sleep is something that has been studied extensively, and results indicate that individuals who sleep either less than seven hours or more than nine hours will increase the potential to get Alzheimer's disease. In addition to the increased potential of getting Alzheimer's disease, poor sleep is tied to heart disease, stroke, Parkinson's, obesity, and diabetes.

We need to realize that the circadian rhythms are different for everyone. I, for example, have always been a morning person.

I have always gone to bed early and risen early. My wife, however, has always been a night owl. Studies indicate that teenagers have a different sleep cycle than adults. This is why most college kids stay up until about two or three in the morning and sleep until noon or one o'clock; this is their natural cycle. Unfortunately, we try to fit them into our schedule. Perhaps this is why many kids doze through many of their morning classes and don't end up learning much from school.

But whether you're up with the roosters or the owls, sleep is a critical component to your health and wellness plan. Your body heals while you rest. During that period, your body gets very little motion, which is one of the reasons that it is important that when you first arise you stretch. Remember to do it correctly to avoid injury.

Making sure that you are not only getting enough sleep, but also good, quality sleep is critical. This is often related to stress. People are not getting good, quality sleep, so they're not entering into a deep sleep cycle. This is what we refer to as rapid eye movement (REM) sleep. We must have at least two to three cycles of good REM sleep to feel refreshed in the morning. If you're not getting into that deep sleep, your body is not healing while you rest.

This deep sleep cycle allows not only your body to heal, but also your mind. Your mind heals as a result of what we commonly refer to as the dreaming process. Dreams give us a mental catharsis. Dreaming allows release of the mental stressors that are eating away at you. This will reduce or remove physical and physiological manifestations of emotional or psychological stress. You will often find that you solve problems or challenges in your life while you sleep. The answers often come to us when our minds are in the fully relaxed state of deep sleep.

The quality of your sleep can be significantly enhanced by using the 31 easy techniques outlined below. Even though they're simple things and some of them may even seem silly, they can have a very positive impact on your sleep cycles.

1. **Determine just how much sleep you need.** You will do this through experimentation. Start on a Friday night or a night that you don't have to be up at a specific time the next day. Go to bed at about the same time as you would on a work night. Do not set your alarm for the next morning. See what time you wake up naturally. Do it again Saturday night. Begin to determine your natural sleep cycle. This will assist you in determining how much sleep your body naturally requires. It is important to realize that your body requires anywhere between 7 and 9 hours of sleep to repair and regenerate. The above exercise will not only help you to determine your natural sleep cycle, but will also let you know if you fall between these parameters of sleep. You may find that if you are sleep deprived you sleep more as you begin this process, but in time, you will find your true sleep hours.

2. **Play with your sleep time.** Once you have completed your research and your perfect sleep time is determined, you can play with it. If you think that you may be getting too much sleep and perhaps are not being as productive as you would like, try cutting 15 minutes off of it. If you find that you are feeling fatigued the next

day, replace the 15 minutes the next night and don't cut back any further on your sleep time.

3. **Give yourself enough time to wake up.** Everyone does this at a different rate. Most people need to give themselves time in their morning ritual to wake up. If you need to use caffeine and other stimulants to wake up, then there is a deeper problem. Your adrenal glands may be fatigued from continued stress that the body is unable to get going without a jolt of caffeine. This is all too common in our fast-paced world.

4. **Fragmented sleep does not supply your body with the deep, restful REM sleep that it requires to rejuvenate and heal itself.** The cumulative effects of the insult to your body can be devastating to your health and wellness. So, do not keep hitting the snooze alarm and think that you are getting more rest. You are not! What you are doing is depriving yourself of healthy, restful sleep. The answer to this dilemma is to get to bed earlier!

5. **Make up for that sleep that you lost.** Every two-hour block of time that you are up and going requires one hour of rest and regeneration time. If you miss out on sleep one night, then get to bed earlier the next night. Yes, Mom was right. Trying to catch up on the weekend is akin to trying to diet just on the weekends and expecting to lose weight.

6. **Napping is allowed, with a few caveats.** First, don't nap for too long. A power nap of 20 minutes to an hour is okay, depending on your age. Just don't do it too

late in the day or you may disturb your sleep cycle for the upcoming night. The latest that you should finish your nap is four o'clock, or else you will probably alter your sleep cycle for the upcoming night. Many people, octogenarians and those even further along in life, will start using naps on a periodic basis because of energy needs and physiological requirements of their bodies. So don't feel bad about napping so long as you're doing it for the right reasons. Many great people—Einstein and Edison—napped regularly, recharging their brains and bodies. But make sure it's not a way of compensating for poor quality sleep, and make sure you're not doing it for too long at a time.

7. **If you must consume caffeine, do not do it after two o'clock.** Don't try to fool yourself on this one. This rule applies to coffee, caffeinated soft drinks, energy drinks, chocolate, and caffeinated tea. Six hours after you take a sip of a caffeinated drink or eat chocolate, you will still have one-half of the ingested caffeine in your body.

8. **No alcohol within three hours of going to bed.** Contrary to the beliefs of many, a drink within three hours of your sleep time will reduce your ability to rest well. Alcohol is metabolized quickly, so a drink with dinner or after work (preferably dry red wine) will generally be out of your system by the time you are ready to go to bed.

9. **You should never smoke, but if you are addicted, then don't smoke before you go to bed.** While you lie awake in bed trying to go to sleep, your body is actually going through a minor withdrawal. You crave another hit.

Nicotine is a much stronger stimulant than caffeine. Needless to say, if you are a smoker you need to stop smoking. You will find that if you smoke two packs of cigarettes a day, when you quit, the time that you lay in bed waiting to go to sleep every night will immediately be cut in half.

10. **Take a walk or run (not too strenuous!) between five and seven o'clock in the evening.** You need to exercise, but it needs to be the right type and at the right time. If you exercise too strenuously at night, you will elevate your core temperature too much. Your core temperature must be reduced before bed to stimulate melatonin production. The best time to exercise is between five and seven o'clock in the evening. Strenuous exercise should be done earlier in the day because your core temperature will remain elevated for five to six hours.

11. **Set the bedroom temperature to 65 degrees.** If you are accustomed to having the temperature in your bedroom too high, it might be the culprit in your challenges with sleep. If you are used to the temperature being too high, you might want to lower the temperature slowly over a period of days. If you feel cool, put an extra blanket on.

12. **Use low lighting in the bedroom.** Remember the bedroom is designed for just two things. Number one is sleep and rest. The other reason that you have a bedroom is so that you and your lover can experience the natural, health-promoting benefits of lovemaking. The act of lovemaking benefits your move right and think right pillars as well. Reduced lighting will produce benefits

in both of these endeavors in your bedroom. The light should produce a gentle, subdued glow. Replacing your 60-watt bulb with a 45-watt or an adjustable three-way bulb would be best.

13. **Use a dimmer.** This will allow you to lower the lighting a little at a time. This will cause a gentle and subtle drowsing effect on your eyes and mind.

14. **Block all secondary light out of the room.** If there is a streetlight that shines in the window even though the curtain is drawn, then try dark, light-blocking curtains. If there is light that comes in through a crack in the bottom of the door, you can shove a towel under the door. You can even use an eye mask to block that secondary light.

15. **Completely block LCD lighting.** That means clocks, TVs, stereos, and DVD and VCR players, along with cell phones and tablets. Turn them off, cover them, or get them out of the room.

16. **Eliminate or mask noise.** A noise of even 60 decibels will stimulate your nervous system and make it difficult for you to get a restful sleep. You can dampen background noise by using a fan set on a low speed or an air purifier, both of which are in place of a more expensive white noise device. A snoring partner can also create a difficult sleeping environment for the individual on the receiving end of the offending auditory insult, so this technique number 16 is an important one for those of you who are experiencing this issue.

17. **Use earplugs or noise-blocking headphones.** Sleeping in a shirt with a breast pocket worn backward with either a tennis ball or a golf ball in the pocket will keep the snuffleupagus off of his or her back. Because most chronic snorers do their best work while on their backs, this technique will force them to move to their side, which will dampen the sound effects.

18. **Decorate your bedroom in restful colors.** The colors of your sleeping area will affect your sleep. You should use light pastel colors with few, if any, bright accent colors. Sedating colors will assist with a restful sleep.

19. **Get the clutter out of your bedroom.** I mean clean it up! The old adage about clutter applies here too, not just to your desk. We don't need a cluttered mind when we are trying to relax and go to sleep. So de-clutter the bedroom. Put some nice plants and pictures in that room to stimulate pleasant dreams.

20. **Replace that worn-out mattress.** Depending on the quality of the mattress that you use, you may need to replace it every 10 years or more frequently. The type of mattress that you choose is a personal preference. You need to go into the showroom and give mattresses a test drive, and I don't mean to lie down for a few minutes and say "I think this one feels okay." No, give it a real test, and if there will be two of you will be sharing the bed, you both need to test it at the same time. Many mattress retailers have a 30- or 90-day return policy. If you decide within the allotted time frame that you don't like it, return it for a replacement. I would also

recommend that you wait for a sale. There is a significant markup on mattresses, and you can often buy one at half price the sticker price if you wait until a sale and do some comparison shopping.

21. **Wear seasonally appropriate bed clothing.** If you need to be a little bit warmer in bed, then it is time for the flannels. Always remember that cotton allows your body to move and breathe better.

22. **Avoid underwear of any type at night.** Truly, the absolute healthiest way to sleep is in your birthday suit. This will allow freedom of movement without binding clothing, which can cause a number of concerns, including blocking blood flow.

23. **Choose the correct neck and head support.** The pillow that you choose must be correct for you and properly support your neck. The one-size-fits-all mentality does not apply here. Look at how people differ; some have thick bull necks, while some have long, elegant necks. The key is that your head is supported in a neutral position. It should not be too high or too low. This applies whether you are a side or back sleeper. (Do not sleep on your stomach because doing so causes undo stress on your lower back and neck.)

24. **Don't forget the importance of comfortable bedding.** Cotton sheets are the best to use because they breathe and are absorbent. Nothing feels better after a long day than climbing into a freshly made bed with clean cotton sheets against your skin.

25. **Remove all of the IT from your sleeping area.** That's right; no laptops, no iPods, no iPads. If you're going to read, use an actual book and not your e-reader. All of these IT products are stimulants to your brain and make it more difficult for your brain and body to shut down, relax, and prepare for proper rest.

26. **Establish and stick to a relaxing pre-sleep routine.** You need to unwind before bed. That may mean taking a bath or shower or reading a light or funny novel. Perhaps it means finishing a task so that your next day starts off fresh, without any tasks to be completed before you can get moving with the activities of the new day. You may want to fold that laundry or clear the mess in the sink or on your desk. Whatever your routine is to relax or clear your mind, just do it every night.

27. **Guard the boudoir.** This one is for parents of young children and is also a rule that, I have to admit, my wife and I are guilty of having broken. Establish a no-kids zone in your bed at night. I know this may seem challenging to those of you whose young children have developed the habit of awakening and running into Mom and Dad's bed for comfort and a restful night's sleep—for them. Generally, this means that the night will be anything but restful for Mom and Dad. It is very difficult to sleep soundly with the sole of a little foot jammed into your ribs or with about six inches of bed between you and the floor. Instead of letting them into your bed, try establishing a sleep zone for the little midnight visitor. This could be a sleeping bag set up on

the floor or a makeshift tent constructed of pillows and blankets in the corner where your child can curl up and get a good night's sleep while Mom and Dad slumber undisturbed.

28. **If you wake up, get up.** Even after applying all of my previous recommendations, if you are having trouble making it through the night and you wake up, then get up. If you wake up and in 15 or 20 minutes you are still awake, go into a different room. Keep the lights low and don't watch TV; do something mundane and boring. Stargaze or read something relaxing, like a daily devotional, the Bible, or the comics in the paper. Don't go on the computer or pick up your iPod or e-reader. In about 15 minutes, you should feel tired again and can get back in bed to enjoy the remainder of the night.

29. **Stretch before you go to bed.** This will not only loosen up those tight muscles and joints, but will also increase circulation to tissues. It is a great preparation for sleep.

30. **Sleep more to lose weight.** By sleeping right, you will assist your body in regulating your weight. If you sleep eight hours a night, you will not gain weight as easily. There will not be as many waking hours in which to shove food into your mouth. Also, when you are tired, your metabolism is off and you tend to eat more to keep you going. So, sleep more and lose weight.

31. **Better sleep will improve your memory.** The brain continues to function while we sleep. For some of us, it may function better than while we are awake. This is the

time when learned behavior becomes solidified into our memory banks. Students need to get enough good sleep to learn, but this also applies to the rest of us. We need to engrain the knowledge we gained the day before into our memories. Improve your memory power by getting enough sleep.

If you begin applying the techniques outlined here, you'll increase both the quality and quantity of your sleep. If sleep is a problem for you, your medical practitioner may prescribe sleep aids, but compensating for a lack of good, quality sleep with sleep aids is not the best way to change in the long term. Every drug has secondary effects, and usually they're negative secondary effects on some other gland, organ, or tissue.

Sometimes sleep aids may be necessary. A lack of sleep will cause negative mental and physiological changes in a relatively short period of time. If you must use some type of a sleep aid, there are many healthier alternatives that can be used, such as tryptophan, which is found in milk. Tryptophan enhances serotonin levels and assists in sleep production. Another alternative is melatonin. Melatonin is a precursor to serotonin; by increasing your melatonin levels, you subsequently increase your serotonin levels, the hormone in your brain that lulls you into sleep. Valerian root is a natural sedative and an alternative to the pharmacopeia of sleep-enhancing drugs.

These are substances that I prefer not to see used, and certainly not on a prolonged basis. This also applies to the nutritional and herbal sleep aid supplements mentioned above. Rather than taking them, try altering your lifestyle and sleep environment. Remember that by increasing your motion and mobility you will increase and enhance your sleep habits as well.

Getting up correctly is important, too, but something many people don't stop to ponder. In my practice, one of the first things I teach my patients is how to get out of bed in the morning. Lie on your side and push yourself up with your elbow on your fist into a seated position as you let your legs drop off of the side of the bed. It keeps your spine straight and your joints less stressed as you arise.

I also give my patients exercises to build into their daily routines. The exercises are simple yoga-type stretches. Bringing both knees to the chest is a simple lower back stretching exercise that releases pain and tension. The pelvic tilt is another good stretching and strengthening exercise. If your sleep surface is firm enough, you can do these exercises just before you get out of bed in the morning, and again just before going to sleep at night.

I also want to touch on the importance of refueling your body properly when you wake up; this is extremely important. All too often, breakfast is something many people forego, usually because they don't feel that they have time. But you've been fasting for eight to nine hours prior to waking up, and your body needs a recharge. That recharge should be good, quality food. There's no problem with eating a high-carb food in the morning in the form of fruits, but don't forget that protein is important too since it keeps you going through the morning. Cereals, which became the craze back in the 1930s and 1940s, are not necessarily the best quality energy source for your body first thing in the morning. Instead, try protein in the form of nut butters (almond or cashew as an example, but not necessarily peanut butter). Eggs are also a great source of protein. For those of you who are not vegetarian or vegan, there's nothing wrong with eating some meat in the morning. I don't necessarily mean highly-processed meats like bacon, but you can eat chicken or turkey or even fish as a breakfast food and that will carry you through the morning better than many of the refined grain-based carbohydrates with which many of you begin your days. They are generally burned up in a short period of time and leave you hungry, tired, and lethargic.

. . . . .

In closing, I would like to remind you that my mission here at the Center and with everything I do when I teach a class or give a seminar, is designed to do one thing, and it is this: "To change humanity by teaching the things that you can do to create a genetically congruent lifestyle that will divert your life path from a sickness and disease paradigm to a health and wellness paradigm." I not only teach these things, but I live and demonstrate them to those around me through my actions and my lifestyle. It's important that I walk the talk, because I know that ultimately, it is important that you follow my example. My goal is to see that you, by learning these things and applying them, will positively affect others. The changes that you make in the way that you live your life will be contagious.

This is how this movement will affect millions of people. You must simply have the strength and desire to do what you need to do in order to generate the changes that I have described. I have seen it happen with thousands of my patients and individuals that I have lectured and spoken to in the past. The changes that occur in your body are going to be observed by others, and the positive feedback that you receive from those around you will motivate you to move further down the road toward health and wellness. You will be an example for others. That's the way I want you to see yourself. Focus on where you are going and do not worry about the criticisms and disturbances that come up in the interim from circumstances, surroundings, and others with whom you interact. These criticisms may be coming from well-intentioned loved ones, coworkers, or acquaintances. When you accomplish this you will get to the point of improved health and wellness. You will then be able to teach others what you now know.

I wish you the best in your quest. I look forward to hearing from you and seeing how you've changed your life and made the progress you have dreamed of by applying these simple principles to your daily routine and lifestyle.

Printed in the USA
CPSIA information can be obtained
at www.ICGtesting.com
JSHW012033140824
68134JS00033B/3042